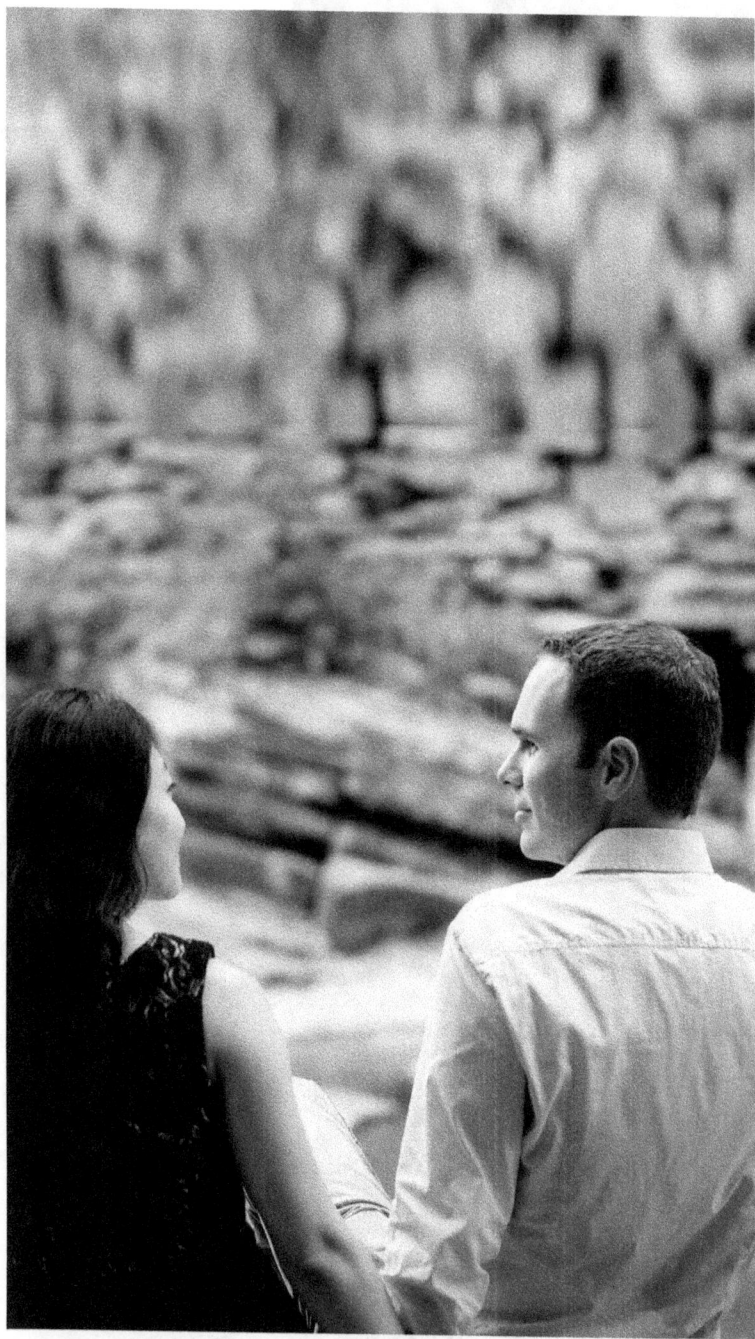

The World's Greatest Weight Loss Secret

How to Convert Your Family to a Gluten-Free, Paleo, or Low-Carb Diet

By *Jeremy Hendon*

First Edition 2014

Table of Contents

PREFACE
— ONE STATISTIC

I care about only one statistic. Just one.

How likely is it that you will be successful in the long run at losing fat and staying healthy?

That statistic is not pretty. At most, 20% of people who lose weight can keep it off for at least a year[1]. That does NOT include people who never lost weight in the first place.

You're lucky. We know more about diet and nutrition than ever before, and you're caring for and nourishing your body by using a Paleo, low-carb, or gluten-free diet.

These diets work. I've seen them work for thousands of people, including myself. Even with the right diet, though, you're still going to be tempted, tired, and find yourself in tough situations that will test your commitment. Your diet is just the beginning.

Here's the world's biggest diet and weight loss secret:

*If you want to be successful long-term, you **must** have the support, encouragement, and involvement of your family and friends.*

Having the support of your family makes you at least 3 times more likely to stick to your diet and maintain your weight-loss over the long term[2].

---

1 / "Long-term weight loss maintenance" Am. J. Clin. Nutr. July 2005, vol. 82 no. 1 222S-225S. http://ajcn.nutrition.org/content/82/1/222S.full

2 / "Benefits of recruiting participants with friends and increasing social support for weight loss and maintenance" Journal of Consulting and Clinical Psychology, Vol 67(1), Feb 1999, 132-138. http://psycnet.apa.org/journals/ccp/67/1/132/

You don't need a statistic to tell you this, because you know that you're less likely to stick to your diet when your family and friends tempt you by keeping junk food around the house or inviting you out to less-than-ideal restaurants. So what can you do?

The answer is simple but not always easy. You must involve your family and friends. Fortunately, this will not only make your diet much more successful, it will also improve your relationships with your family and friends in ways you never imagined.

So get ready. If you're interested in improving your health while also strengthening your family and your relationships, then you're going to love this book.

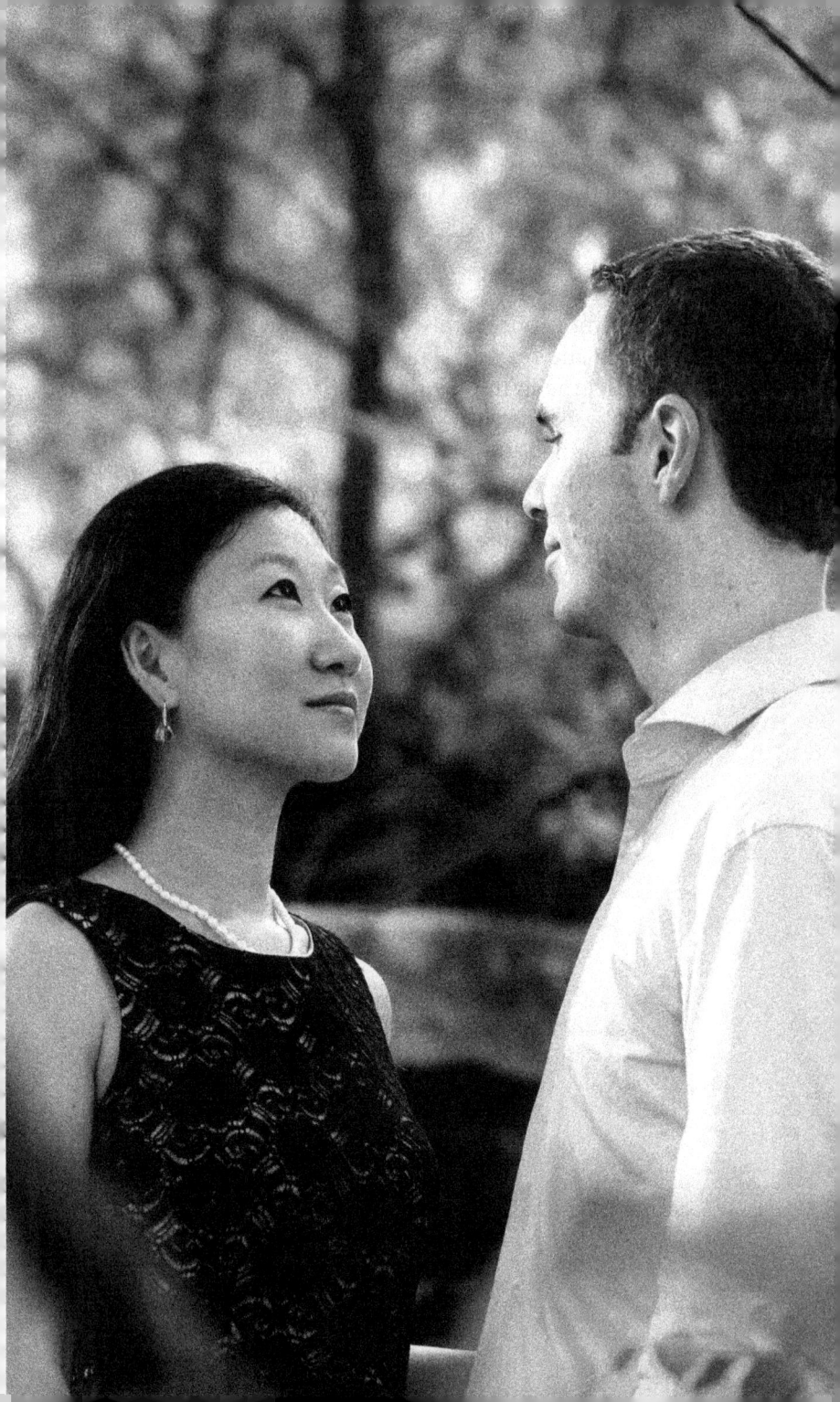

INTRODUCTION
— THE SECRET I LEARNED THE HARD WAY

Have you ever wondered how much easier it would be if your entire family was *EXCITED* about making healthier food, exercise, and lifestyle choices? What if all of your friends were also on board?

How easy would it be for you to make better choices and decisions about what you eat if you had the unflinching support of your family and friends?

Getting healthy, losing weight, exercising, or sticking to any sort of diet – these tasks are difficult in the best of circumstances. They are far harder if you're unable to count on the support of your spouse, your partner, your kids, and your friends.

If you think about it, then you <u>probably already know</u> all of this. Not enough support is one of the biggest things standing in the way of you getting healthier. Even so, most of us spend no time or energy planning for how to get that support.

I want to assure you that it is not only *possible* to gain the support of your friends and family (and eventually convert them) I've actually seen *thousands* of people do it.

And many of these people have been exactly where you probably are (and where I was). They started out thinking that their families were *too stubborn, too unsupportive,* or just *too lazy* to even care.

Everybody's situation is slightly different. However, you can use the same approach as thousands of successful folks in order to get your own family excited about eating and living healthier. Believe it or not, you can get them excited about a gluten-free, Paleo, or low-carb diet.

There's a formula for how to do it, and that's what I'm going to show you in this book.

HOW BEING FAT MADE ME TERRIBLE AT RELATIONSHIPS

My wife, Louise, is a very successful author, blogger, and speaker (predominantly on health and food-related topics), and she runs one of the magazines that we own (Healthy Recipes Magazine).

You might be thinking, "Wow, Jeremy is really lucky to have found someone who is so excited about health and food."

And I am extremely lucky. Louise is amazing.

However, for the first 7 years of our relationship, I didn't know anybody who was less interested in nutrition, health, and diet than Louise. She'd never been overweight, and even though she had a few health issues, she was completely unmotivated to change her diet or lifestyle.

On the other hand, I had always been the fat kid. I spent my entire life hating that I was fat and trying to get in better shape. It has always been a very personal issue for me.

When I was 7 years old, I remember wondering why I couldn't run as fast as all the other kids. That is one of the first times I remember feeling fat, but it certainly wasn't the last or the most painful memory. Throughout high school and college, I rarely dated anybody because I was so uncomfortable with my own body that I was sure nobody else could possibly like me.

In retrospect, I realize that I saw myself in a much worse way than how other people saw me. **However, because I believed that I was too fat, my attitude continually stood in the way of me developing meaningful relationships.** (I'll tell you below how this realization has completely changed the way I now approach diet and health.)

It took me a long time to realize that focusing on my relationships might actually improve my success at losing weight.

I HAVEN'T ALWAYS BEEN A GREAT HUSBAND

By the time I met Louise, I had lost some weight, but I was still struggling. No matter how hard I exercised or dieted, I inevitably gained back most or all of the fat that I'd lost.

About 4 years after I met Louise, I decided to radically clean up the way I ate and commit to a Paleo diet. A lot of my friends and coworkers told me that I was being too extreme or that it wouldn't work, but it turned out to be one of the best decisions I've ever made.

Sticking to that decision was far tougher than I imagined it would be, and many times I thought about just giving up all together. One of the toughest things is that Louise spent several years resenting my new diet and commitment to exercise, and she often tried to talk me out of it.

Louise has always been very supportive of me, but that doesn't mean that she has liked every decision that I've made. *Far from it.* (I've made a lot of mediocre and bad decisions that I won't get into.)

Cleaning up my diet and lifestyle was an excellent decision, but I approached it in the worst possible way.

When I made the decision to clean up my diet and change how I ate, I didn't include Louise at all in that decision. I didn't ask her what she thought about the decision – and worse, I didn't even invite her to help me.

Rather, I simply *informed* her that I was going to start eating differently, and that she could eat the same way as me or she could eat whatever food she wanted to buy/prepare/cook. Louise didn't act mad – in fact, she *seemed* ok with it. At least I *thought* she seemed ok with it – I was actually ignoring some very obvious signs to the contrary.

As time went along, I realized that she was getting angrier and angrier that we were often not even eating together and that I was essentially forcing her to eat the food that I was cooking (which, admittedly, wasn't very imaginative or flavorful at that time).

If anybody told you that you could either do things their way or else fend for yourself, then you would probably react negatively and defensively to that sort of proposition.

So it's no wonder that Louise reacted less than enthusiastically.

The way I approached changing my diet was a bad way to implement any change, much less one that dramatically affected the person I was living with. If you want to have success in your own diet and in your own relationships, then please don't start out the way I did.

HOW I BECAME A MUCH BETTER HUSBAND

Louise and I had MANY fights over food. And I'm not exaggerating when I say that it lasted for years.

Today, however, Louise believes in the changes to our diet and lifestyle at least as much as I do. And that's not because I pressured her for long enough.

I distinctly remember lying in bed one night and finally telling Louise *three things* that I'd never told her before:

1. I told her **why it was so important to me** to change my diet and try to lose weight. I explained what it meant to me.

2. I told her **why her support was incredibly important to me.** I explained how her support was the thing that made everything easier for me, as well as more pleasant.

3. I asked her if she could help me out in a few specific ways. Literally, I asked for 5 things that I knew she could do to help me out.

Not everything changed the next day, but a lot did. It required several more conversations, and it wasn't solely a result of me telling her what was important to me. She also started telling me specifically what would make everything easier for her.

Within a month, though, we stopped fighting over food and diet. And within a year after that, Louise was fully committed to a diet that she thought for years was crazy.

Since that time, it's been easier than ever for me to eat healthy and live a lifestyle that nourishes my body. More importantly, though, Louise and I are happier than ever.

THE MISSING PIECE OF THE PUZZLE

For much of my life, I thought that being fat stood in the way of great relationships for me. I felt like I needed to lose fat and look better before I could improve my relationship.

As it turns out, improving my relationship and my communication was the key ingredient for improving my diet and health.

And changing my diet and lifestyle was actually the perfect opportunity to improve my relationship.

For years, I blamed Louise for making it harder for me to stick to my diet. Ironically, I also felt like I was imposing on her. It seemed like Louise always had to give in to whatever restaurant I wanted to go, just because my diet was more limiting.

For instance, because I felt like I was imposing on her, I'd always apologize for forcing her go to the restaurants that I wanted to go to. And while apologizing can be a good thing, it continually made Louise feel like she was getting the raw end of the deal. It made her feel like she had no say – like she was powerless in those situations and in our relationship.

And I'm not the only one who felt this way. I've talked to thousands of people who have the exact same sentiment. You likely have felt one or both of those feelings in your own life.

Several years ago, Louise and I founded 2 health

websites and 2 health magazines that are all now very successful. We receive dozens and sometimes hundreds of daily emails from people who are either thanking us for helping them or else asking us for help or advice on problems.

Trying to convert or gain the support of family is the most commonly mentioned obstacle. This is the #1 issue that someone starting a gluten-free, Paleo, or low-carb diet faces. And if you believe statistics or even just thousands of stories, it's one of the keys to long-term success.

Fortunately, it's an obstacle that can be overcome and that can change your life in ways that you've never imagined.

THE 3-STEP PROCESS THAT WILL CHANGE YOUR LIFE AND YOUR BODY

Imagine a situation in which your spouse, partner, or children feel like they're empowered. Imagine them deciding that they want to help and support you.

This might sounds like a small difference or it might even sound impossible, but I promise that empowering your spouse, partner, and/or kids is neither insignificant nor impossible.

I've written this book because I've seen so many people either succeed or fail based on the way that they deal with their family. I had my own experience, but seeing how thousands of other people deal with it has been invaluable.

And I'm not bragging, but I don't think anybody else out there is getting the same results that I'm getting. I certainly can't claim to solve 100% of situations, but my approach truly works whenever someone consistently applies it.

It worked for me before I even knew what I was doing, but by helping many other people in this situation, I've refined and improved the process.

Getting your family on board with major diet and health changes (whether gluten-free, Paleo, or low carb) is a simple 3-step process:

1. You must change the way that you think about diet and health as it relates to your relationship with your family. As I'll explain in Chapter 2, you must stop viewing it as a hindrance or imposition and start viewing it as a **golden opportunity** to improve and enhance your relationships.

2. You must get extremely clear and specific in your own mind (and on paper) as to how your family can best help and support you. If you skip this step, then you'll forever be frustrated, and so will your family. I explore this concept in Chapter 3.

3. You must commit to regular conversations with your family. Your family is not a "problem" that you deal with once and everything is fixed. In fact, it's not a "problem" at all. It's an ever-evolving relationship that can either support you or drag you down, and the choice is yours. Chapter 4 is all about how to have these conversations.

The process is simple, but that does not mean it's easy or without effort. It takes work, and it can take time. But the results are worth it.

My life has changed dramatically because of the ways I've learned to communicate with and involve Louise, and I know that you can achieve the same. This book will help you get there.

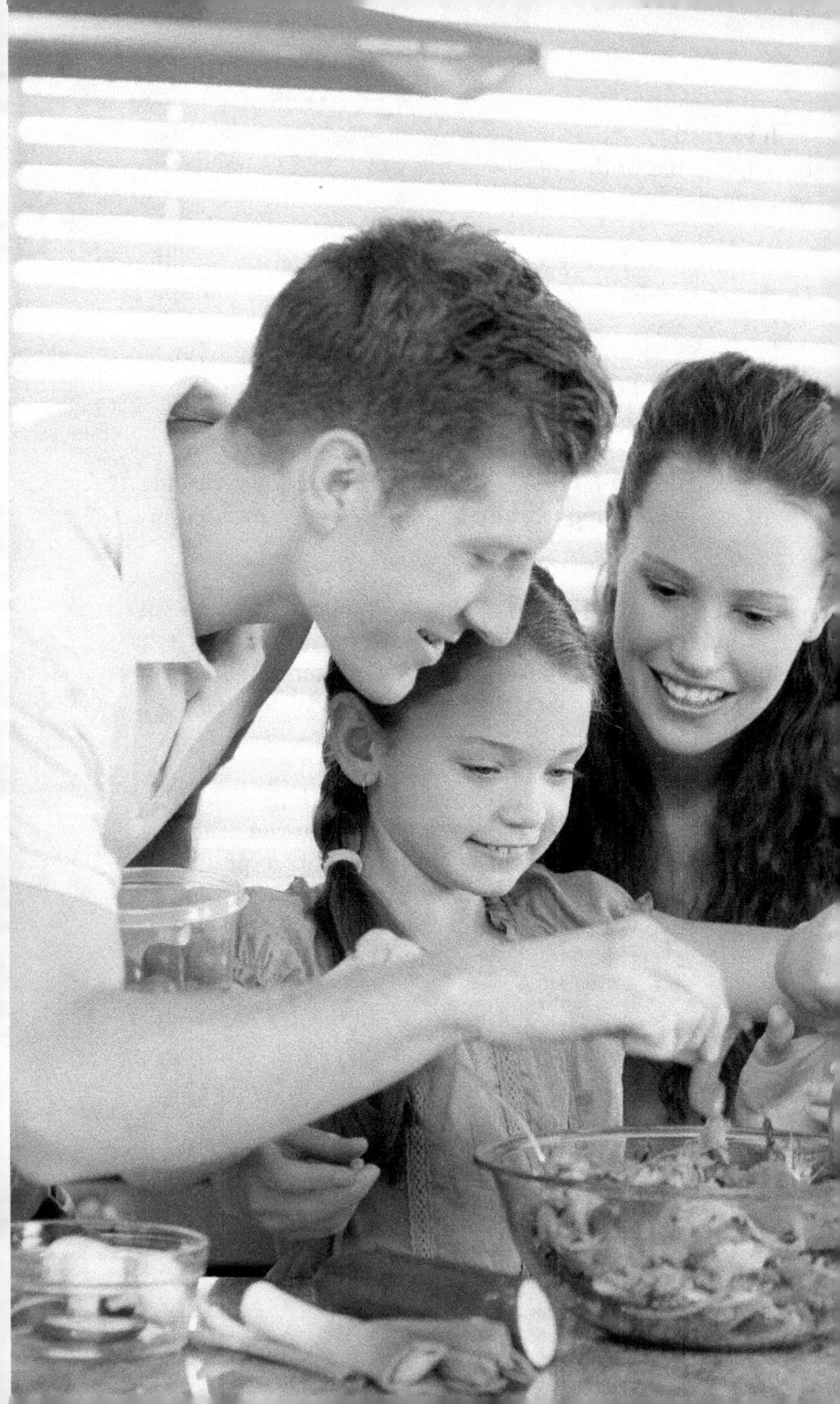

CHAPTER 1:
IS YOUR FAMILY STUBBORN?

Do you ever feel like, by changing your diet or committing to a healthier lifestyle, you're becoming *a burden* on your friends and family? Like you're forcing them to *accommodate* your new way of life?

Or maybe you're disappointed that your stubborn spouse, partner, or kids don't give you *more support*? Do you wish that they'd simply *stop tempting you* and stubbornly refusing to improve their own diets and health?

Every day, I talk to people who are dealing with similar situations and issues. One woman's husband teases her every day about her diet. Another man has two teenage kids who bring home junk food every day and encourage him to eat it. Another woman feels like she's burdening her supportive family by no longer feeding them the junk food that they've always loved.

I could list hundreds of other examples, and I'm sure your situation is a little bit different than every one of them. However, being in a situation like this is the rule rather than the exception.

Thousands of people have successfully gained the support of their family and friends, and you can have the same success if you start with the *right intent.*

However, you're going to need to radically change the way that you view the entire situation. As I'll explain in Chapter 2, you must view your diet, your health, and your lifestyle as a *golden opportunity* to connect with your family and to actually improve those relationships.

If you can fundamentally shift the way that you approach your family on this subject, then you'll get more support and be more successful than you ever imagined. And in the process, you'll dramatically improve your relationship with your spouse/partner and kids.

It sounds incredible, but I truly see dietary change as an opportunity to not only get comfortable with yourself and your body but also to *improve every single relationship in your life.*

Unfortunately, most of us (including myself for a very long time) royally mess it up.

THE 4 PROBLEM WAYS WE TYPICALLY TALK TO OUR FAMILIES

Getting the support of your spouse, partner, and/or children can make eating well and exercising both easy and fun. Ideally, you would also like to help them eat and live a little bit healthier. You can't accomplish any of that unless you approach the issue with the proper intent and with a positive mindset.

For example, I often get angry at Louise for running late or not being on time. And because I'm angry, it doesn't really matter what I say – she senses that I'm angry, and she instinctively reacts by getting defensive and not wanting to cooperate. However, if I tell her beforehand how important it is for us to get to a particular event on time (before I'm angry), then she's incredibly more likely to try to be ready early.

The mindset that you have when you talk to your family matters at least as much as the words you use.

If you want your family to support a new way of eating, to support a different form of exercise or physical activity, or even to support you just getting more sleep, then you need to be in the right state of mind to ask for their help.

However, when it comes to the issue of diet and health, most of us approach family in one of four ways, all of which prevent us from succeeding before we even start:

1. We often talk to our family as if they <u>don't care</u> about us or our problems.

Have you ever asked your spouse/partner or kids, "Why'd you do that?" Or maybe you thought to yourself, "Obviously, they don't care about what I want or what's good for me."

We've all had these thoughts at one time or another. We tell ourselves that our situation or problems never cross their mind.

Many people who start a diet (gluten-free, Paleo, low-carb, or otherwise) ask their families, "Why would you buy those cookies and bring them home when you know I'm trying to eat better?" Or maybe they say, "If you really care about me, then you wouldn't always give me such a hard time about not eating junk food."

In each case, we start with the assumption that our spouse and/or kids don't actually care about what we value. And if you start by believing this, then your spouse and/or kids will have less incentive to actually care. Subconsciously, they'll feel like you don't value any of the things that they do to help you or support you, and that will discourage them from doing more to show that they care.

2. We often talk to our family as if they <u>don't understand</u> our problems.

This is a little different than imagining that our family

doesn't care. In this situation, we tell ourselves that they simply don't comprehend what we're going through.

In the past, I have started conversations with Louise by saying, "You don't understand this, but…." None of those conversations ended well.

And any time that you're trying to explain the situation to your spouse or kids, you're trying because you think that they don't understand what you're going through.

Often, when someone starts a new diet or exercise plan, they'll tell their spouse or partner, "I know that you don't understand how hard it is for me to lose weight, but I really need for you to help me out by not tempting me." Or

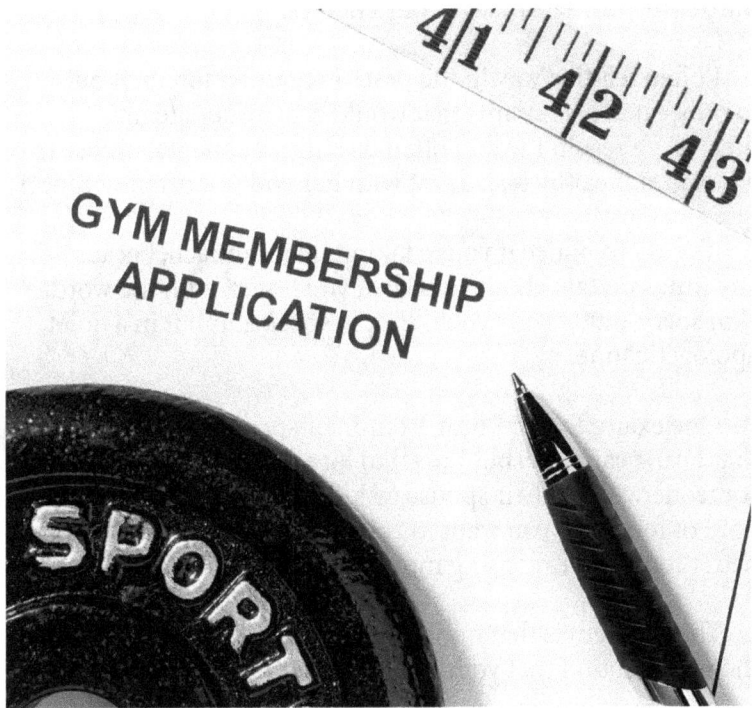

sometimes they'll say, "I know you're not worried about eating better, but it's really important to me."

In both cases, you assume that your spouse/partner doesn't understand how hard it is or why it's important. The problem is that nobody likes admitting that they don't understand, so when you approach your family this way, they're going to shut down mentally and not even try to understand where you're coming from.

3. We often talk to our family as if we are <u>imposing</u> on them.

In the first 2 situations, we feel angry that our family doesn't care about us or understand our situation. Many times, though, we actually feel apologetic, as if we're burdening our family with our choices.

I often felt this way in the past. I regretted forcing Louise to only eat at restaurants that would accommodate my diet. (As a result, I would often use this as a mental excuse to go to an unhealthy restaurant with her and just eat junk food.)

It's easy to notice if you're taking this approach, because any time you talk about your diet, you'll start with the words "I'm sorry, but…." Or you'll simply speak about it in a quiet, apologetic tone.

One example that I hear from many people is "I'm sorry that I can't eat there, but I need to lose some weight." Or often, someone will tell their spouse or kids, "I know this is not the kind of food that you want to eat, but we need to start eating better food and exercising more."

The problem is that underneath all of these statements is the presumption that your diet and your health choices are a burden or hassle for your family. In fact, you might believe this right now. (Don't worry, I'm going to give you specific steps in Chapter 2 to change this belief.)

When you start with this presumption (that you and your choices are a burden), it's practically inevitable that your family is going to also feel like your diet and your health choices are a burden. And if they feel that way, they're not very likely to support or encourage you.

4. We often talk to our family as if they don't matter.

Maybe you think you don't do this. I'd like to believe that. But we all do it to some degree.

For example, have you ever told your kids or spouse, "From now on, I'm not going to eat any [insert your choice of food]?" Or maybe you've told them "I don't care if you keep eating junk, but I'm going to start cooking better food that you can either eat or not eat."

If you ever tell your family about a decision you've made

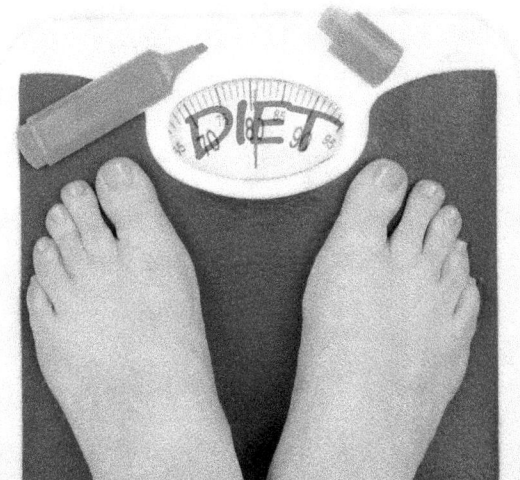

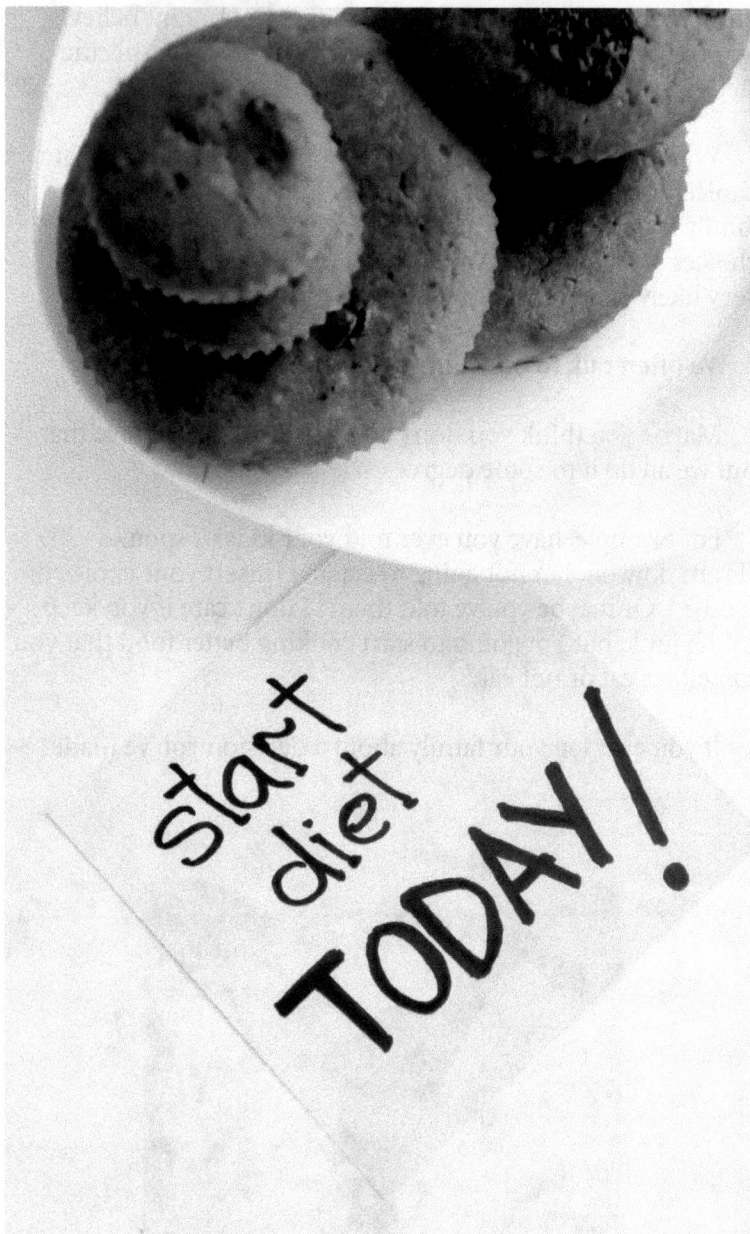

or about a change that you're going to make – unless you first involved them in the decision or asked for their input - then you're adopting the mindset that they don't matter. You've approached the situation as if their input is irrelevant.

If you're telling your family about a diet or health decision you've made, then they are not invested at all in that decision. And because they're not invested, it matters much less to them whether you stick to that decision or succeed at reaching your goal.

YOU WILL NEVER BE PERFECT

You will never fully avoid thinking in one of these four ways. Nobody is perfect, and I still catch myself falling into these traps.

But you need to recognize these approaches and mindsets because they will keep you from seizing your golden opportunity.

You have very little chance of getting the full support of your family if you view them as not caring, not understanding, not mattering, or if you view yourself as a burden. Their support starts with you re-framing the way you view your own dietary and health changes.

Over the next 3 chapters, we'll explore the exact steps involved in implementing the 3-step process that will get your family involved in the best way possible. But if you recognize yourself approaching the issue in any of the 4 problem ways, then you need to stop and step back. You might need some time – whether a few hours or even a few days – to change the way that you think about your diet and how it relates to your family.

When you do take time to step back, then you open up a world of possibilities. Now, let's talk about what to do next.

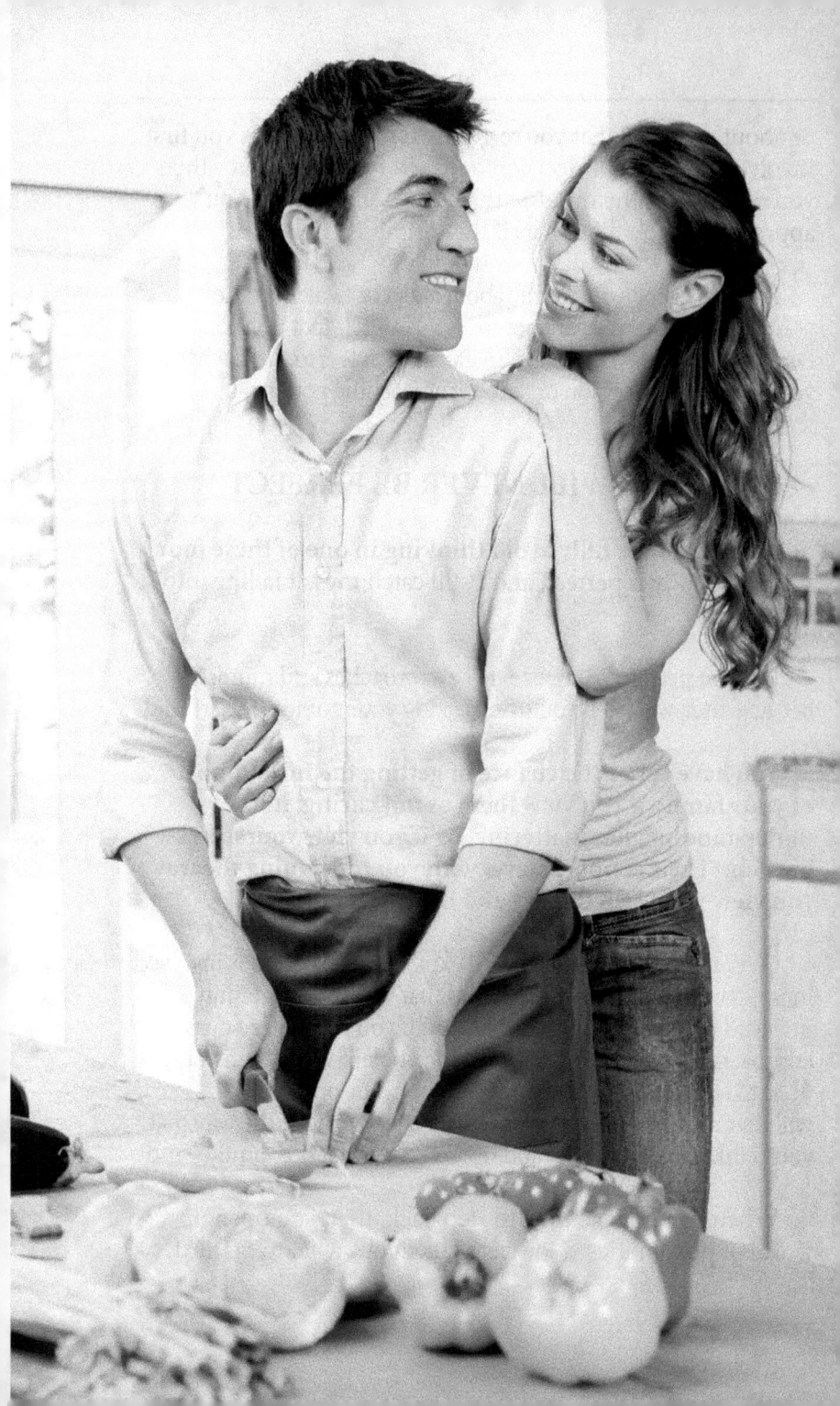

CHAPTER 2:
CLAIM YOUR GOLDEN OPPORTUNITY

Although every person's situation is different, there's one thing that every situation has in common:

If you want to truly gain the support and encouragement of your spouse and/or kids, you MUST view your diet and lifestyle changes as your <u>golden opportunity</u> to IMPROVE your relationship with them.

Think about that for a moment.

I'm not asking you to improve your relationship so that you'll be better able to stick to your diet or to get your family to eat better. *I'm asking you to use your commitment to getting healthier as a way to improve your relationship.*

Right now, your relationship with your spouse and children might be perfect or it might be terrible. Most likely, it's somewhere in between. I know very few people who wouldn't like to make their relationships with their kids, spouse, partner, and the rest of their family better.

This is your chance.

Right now, you probably think that you're forcing them to do or eat something they don't want. And if you feel like that, then how do you think they probably feel?

The answer, of course, is that if you feel like a burden, then they're also going to view your diet as a burden on them.

On the other hand, what if you approached your diet and lifestyle as an opportunity to make life better for your spouse and kids? Imagine feeding them more delicious food and constantly making them physically feel better. Would it still seem like a burden for them?

Perhaps most importantly of all, imagine giving them the *opportunity* to feel more valued and more meaningful. If you could give them that sort of opportunity, how do you think they'd react?

EVERYBODY WANTS TO FEEL VALUED AND MEANINGFUL

This is a universal yearning. We all want to know that we're important, that our lives mean something, and that somebody values what we do.

And when it comes to your spouse, your partner, your kids, and the rest of your family, these feelings are extra-strong.

Unfortunately, we often forget just how strong of a yearning this is. I see this over and over again when someone is trying to get the support of their spouse/partner or kids for a diet or lifestyle change. I'm as guilty as anybody else in this regard.

Quite often, we imagine that our spouse/partner or kids have terrible motives, when it's usually a simple lack of participation, value, and meaning.

For instance, you might tell yourself that your spouse or partner is stubborn or not supportive when he or she refuses to help cook or buys junk food. In actuality, your spouse/ partner likely doesn't feel a part of the process at all and they don't feel like their participation is valuable or meaningful.

Take this example from my own life:

I have never been good at washing the dishes as quickly as

Louise would like. Maybe I was a little bit lazy, but mostly I had different priorities. I always planned on washing the dishes, but more important things came up to delay it.

Louise, of course, didn't view it this way. She believed that I didn't care about helping her out and that I expected her to always wash the dishes.

This became a big argument between us on many days. She'd get mad at me for not washing the dishes, and I'd get mad that she was mad, since I was still planning on washing them, just not yet. These sorts of arguments got us nowhere.

Eventually, though, I started washing the dishes sooner. And it wasn't a result of her yelling at me. It was a result of Louise actually sitting down with me one day and

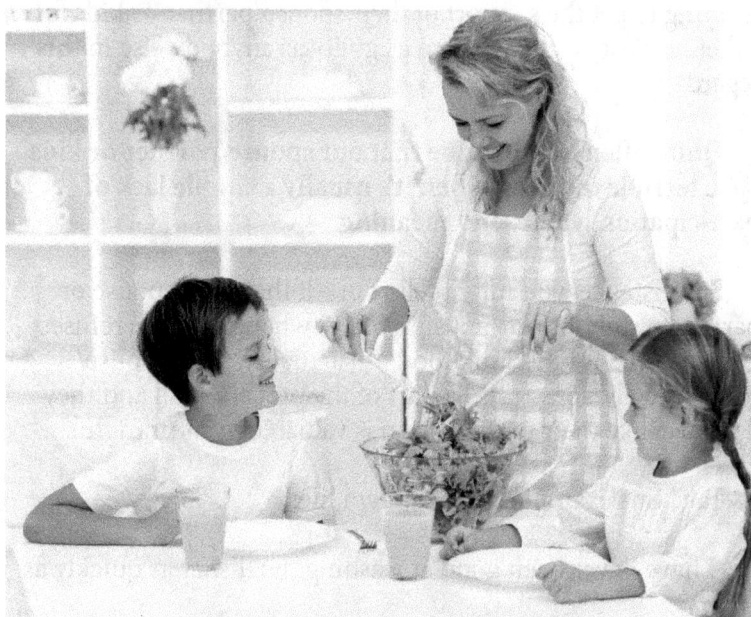

explaining how I could really help her out in terms of her stress level by doing a few things. And she had a few very specific things in mind, one of which was washing dishes as soon as they got dirty.

What changed everything is that Louise started approaching the entire situation differently. She chose to view the situation as an opportunity to let me help her manage her stress level. And once she explained it to me that way, I was incredibly more willing to do whatever I could to help her.

I suddenly felt like my actions (a simple action like washing the dishes more quickly) had a lot more meaning and value.

This is not an excuse for me failing to help out more in the first place. But it's important to remember that the issue of blame simply keeps us from taking steps to make the situation better.

I use the example of washing the dishes because it's easy to understand, and it's also the type of situation that most of us have dealt with, whether with our spouse/partner or our children.

I want you to have a different experience and a different result. I want you to be wildly successful at both eating well and at strengthening your relationship with your family. I'm 100% sure that you can do both, and here's why…

When it comes to your diet and health, your family simply wants to feel valued, meaningful, and helpful.

It may not seem like it right now, but your family wants you to be healthy. They want you to be happy. And given the chance, they would love to help you succeed.

Sometimes a family member will really surprise you and step up without you ever asking. But most of the time, they need an invitation.

YOU MUST GIVE YOUR FAMILY THE OPPORTUNITY TO HELP YOU

As I mentioned above, your family craves the opportunity – just like every other human – to be valuable and to know that their actions and lives have meaning.

They may not be ready yet to change their own bodies and their own diets. That's fine. You're not going to try to convert them yet, but you will be much better off if you *ALLOW* them to help you. And "allow" is a big word here, because that's the only thing stopping anyone from helping you.

Think about every time that a close friend or family member has honestly and genuinely asked you for help. How many times have you turned them down, unless it just wasn't possible for you to help?

Probably almost never.

When someone who you care about asks for your help, you'll most likely do as much as possible in order to make sure that they succeed. There are certainly exceptions – some people won't help out no matter what – but those people are much rarer than you think. Most people just need to be given the opportunity.

You must envision your diet and health changes as a chance to give your family the opportunity to help you.

So far, I've been discussing how to change your mindset in a very abstract way. It's one thing to say that you must view your diet or lifestyle change as a golden opportunity to improve your relationships with your family.

I want to make everything much more concrete.

HOW TO SEIZE YOUR GOLDEN OPPORTUNITY

You must convince yourself that your diet and improved health is going to benefit your family in multiple ways.

It doesn't matter whether you're changing your diet to become gluten-free, Paleo, or low-carb, or if you're just deciding to exercise more. In every case, you must be sure that it's going to benefit your family.

And it really doesn't matter how you convince yourself of this. However, I have found again and again that changing the way you approach your diet and your family starts by being very clear about the ways that your family will benefit.

Hopefully, you already think that getting healthier is good for both you and your family, but you must believe it on a deeper level, and you must remind yourself constantly. The best way to do this is to take some time, write down the ways that your diet will benefit your family, and then revisit those reasons every morning.

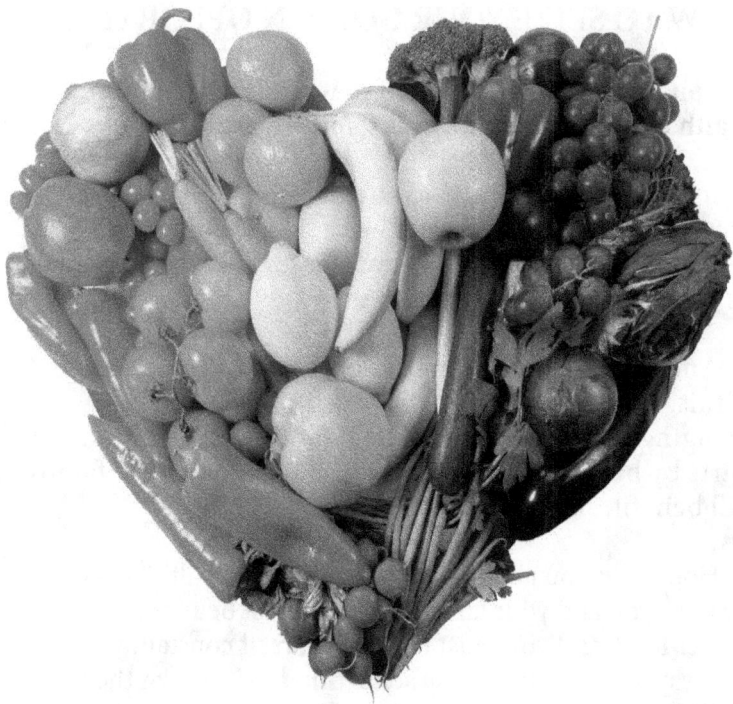

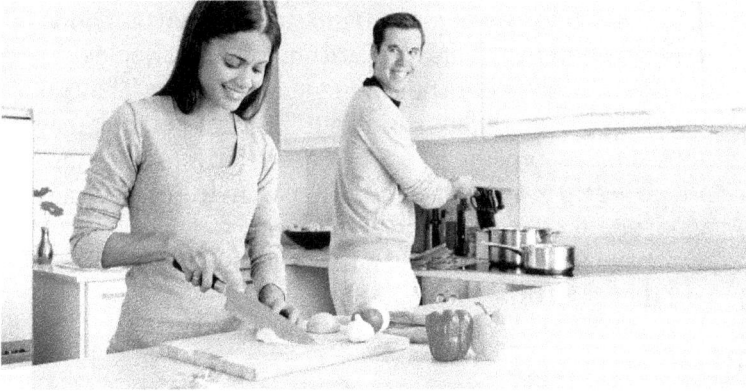

ACTION STEP #1:
Spend 10 minutes writing down all of the reasons that changing your diet and getting healthier will benefit both you AND your family. Put this piece of paper next to your bed and read it every morning.

To get you started, here are several possible reasons that your improved diet and health might benefit your family:

    a. You will be happier. When you eat better, it will make you feel better and put you in a better mood. And this is a great benefit to anyone (your family) who spends a lot of time around you, since we tend to be happiest when the people around us are also happier.

    b. Your family will be healthier. This is something that your spouse or kids may not immediately believe, and it's not your job to convince them. But by changing your own diet and lifestyle, you'll affect theirs by example and by making healthy foods more convenient and available for them. Even if they only eat 5% healthier, that's still an improvement that is a direct result of you changing your own diet and lifestyle.

c. Your family will get a chance to be important and make a difference. This is critical and often overlooked, but if you involve your spouse and kids, then they'll have a chance to make a difference in your life. I know that it may not seem like something they're looking for, but you're just not giving them enough credit. They want to be important, and if you succeed at feeling better, losing weight, or whatever it is you're after, then they will also be proud of the part they played.

You can come up with your own reasons, but it helps to really take time to think about them and then to write them down.

It is critical that you keep these benefits in mind, because you must believe that the change you're making is good for your family also. (And it is, I assure you.) If you start from the opposite assumption, then you'll never give them the opportunity to help you succeed.

And if your family doesn't have the opportunity to help you succeed, then they won't have any reason to try.

TRUST IN THE PROCESS

Asking for help is neither a form of weakness nor a burden. As humans, we get enjoyment, pleasure, and meaning out of helping people we care about.

If you're not willing to ask for the help of your family, then not only are you not going to get the help that you need, but you're denying them a lot of enjoyment, pleasure, and meaning.

You can't perfect either your relationships or your health with a single process, but you need to start somewhere. There's no better place to start than with this 3-step process that has proved to help thousands of dieters.

The process starts by getting in touch with the reasons your diet will help your family. That's step #1 above. Chapters 3 and 4 are all about the next 2 steps in the process.

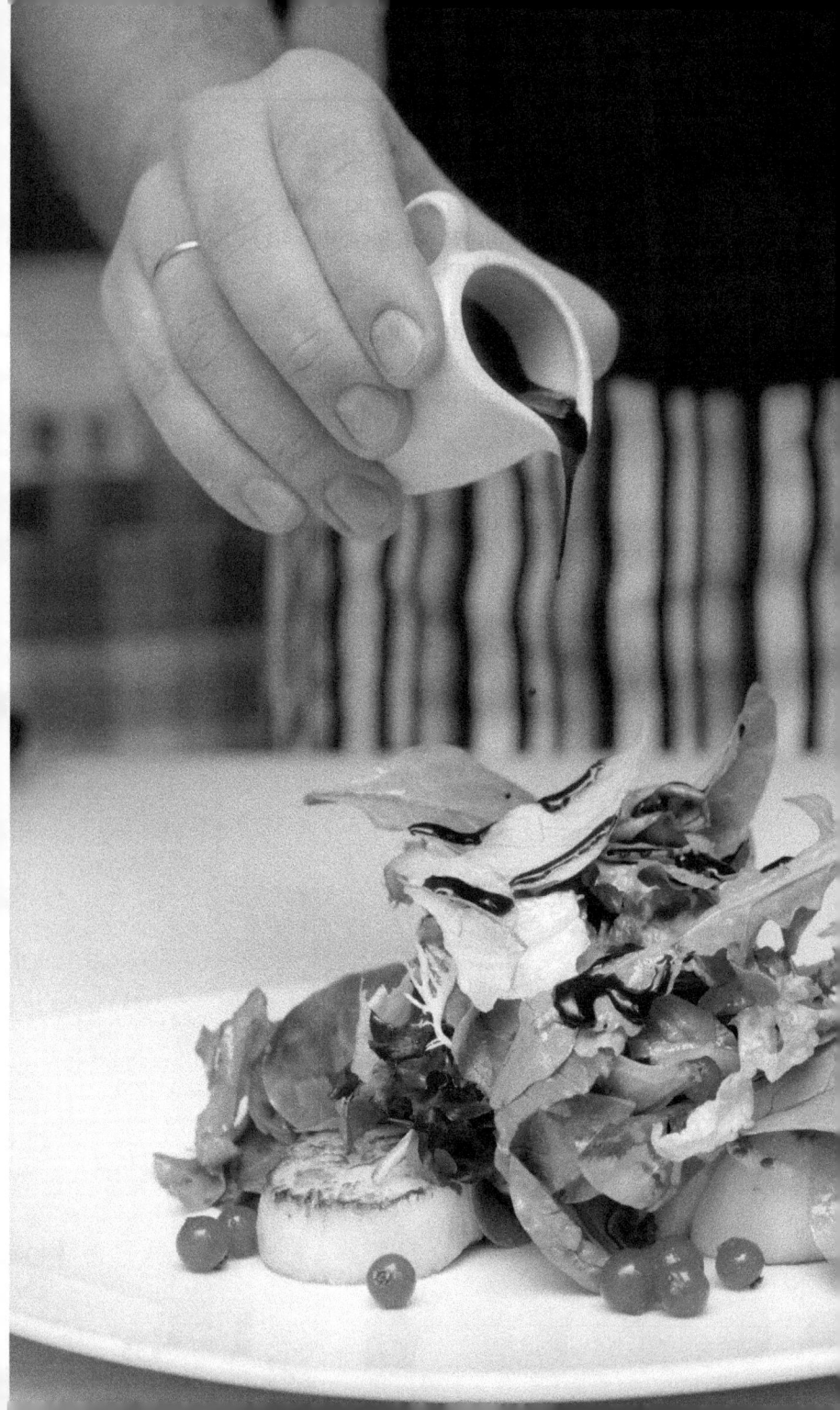

CHAPTER 3:
BE VERY CLEAR ABOUT HOW YOUR FAMILY CAN HELP YOU

By far, the hardest part about getting your family on board is starting with the right intent and the right reasons.

So if you can master the concepts we discussed in Chapter 2 – namely, viewing your diet and lifestyle change as a golden opportunity to improve your relationships with your spouse/ partner and/or children – then you'll be 95% of the way toward getting your family's full support and encouragement.

In fact, if you take nothing else from this book, I'd be extremely happy if you became a little bit more aware of whether you envision your diet and lifestyle change as a hindrance or as an opportunity. This one tiny change in mindset can set you on the path toward dramatically improving your relationships, and it can also make it much more likely that you'll be able to stick to your diet and lifestyle changes.

YOU MUST BE VERY SPECIFIC IF YOU WANT TO TRULY GET YOUR FAMILY ON BOARD

Just as a reminder, seizing your golden opportunity consists of 3 steps:

1. You must start thinking about diet and health as your golden opportunity for improving your relationship with your family.

2. You must get extremely clear and <u>specific</u> in your own mind (and on paper) as to how your family can best help and support you.

3. You must commit to <u>regular conversations</u> with

your family.

If changing your mindset will get you 95% of the way there, then the last 5% involves knowing how your family can help you and having the appropriate conversations.

In Chapter 4, I'm going to guide you step-by-step through having the right conversations with your family. Before we get to that, this chapter will cover how to come up with a plan of ways that your family can help you.

The reason that you're coming up with a plan is not so that you can impose it on your family. The reason you need a plan is because you need to know which areas you need help in, and you need to have a direction (but not an end goal) for your conversations.

Let me explain with an example.

Shortly after I started a Paleo diet, Louise and I moved to New York City. In New York City, at least among our friends, it's accepted that you'll eat out pretty much 7 days per week. After all, nobody wants to be stuck in their 400 square foot apartment, much less cook in it.

Partially because we ate at restaurants so often, I was having a very hard time sticking to my diet. I'd do OK for a week or 2, but then I'd go off the rails for a couple weeks. As a result, I was constantly frustrated and often complained to Louise about my inability to stick to my diet.

Unsurprisingly, Louse quickly got tired of hearing me complain. And I fully realized this. But I had a problem. **I didn't know how to ask Louise for help, because I didn't have any specific idea of how she *could* help.** Even if I'd had

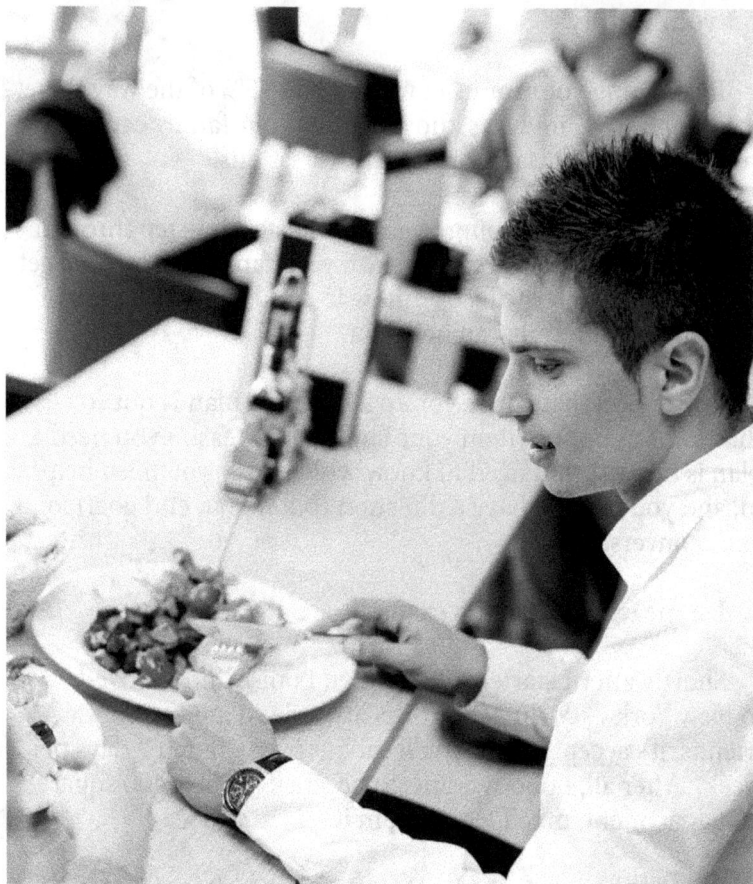

the right mindset, I had no idea *how* to get her to help me.

So I thought about it for a very long time. And eventually, I realized that there were 2 major reasons I wasn't very good at sticking to my diet. First, the restaurants we ate at had very few good, healthy (Paleo) options. Second, I rarely got enough sleep, so I was more likely to make bad choices during the day.

In retrospect, those things should have been obvious to me,

but I simply thought I was bad at sticking to my diet. And until I honed in on my specific problems, I was clueless about how anybody – even Louise – might be able to help me.

WITH CLARITY COMES GREAT POWER

Once I knew what my primary obstacles were, it suddenly became clear to me how Louise might be able to help me.

Unfortunately, I wasn't yet very good at the conversation piece of the puzzle – discussed in the next chapter – that came later, but even without that piece, it was much easier for me to ask for help and start getting her support.

You need to be extremely clear about how your spouse and/or children can support and help you. In particular, you need to know what your obstacles are.

It's nice to think that your family might be able to read your mind and help you in whatever way you need on any given day. For instance, maybe on Tuesday, you need to be comforted after a bad day and encouraged to skip the ice cream. And maybe on Saturday, you need your kids not to bring home the junk food that they decided to buy that day.

I hate to break it to you, but your family will not always know how to best support your diet and lifestyle changes, and they're never going to be able to read your mind.

That doesn't mean that they don't want to support you or that they won't be proud of your accomplishments.

ACTION STEP #2:
Before you talk to your spouse/partner or kids, WRITE DOWN the SPECIFIC things that you need help with.

Please don't try to make this up as you talk to your family. Sit down before you talk to them and come up with a short list of things that would really help you over the next couple months.

For instance, if I were talking to Louise about it, this might be my list:

1. Help keep the house clear of junk foods that most tempt me (ice cream, potato chips, and cookies/crackers).

2. Help choose restaurants that have at least a couple appealing options that are in line with my diet.

3. Help get to bed in time to get 8 hours of sleep every night.

4. At the end of every day, ask me how well I've stuck to my diet. *This is a particularly good thing to ask for, because it helps keep you accountable and shows your spouse or child that you want them to play a role.*

Your list could be entirely different. I can think of a thousand ways that your spouse or kids could help you. Maybe you want 2 hours of their time every Sunday to help you cook food that will last for the rest of the week. Or perhaps it would really help if they let you block off an hour of time every day to exercise or go to the gym.

Whatever your list is, it should be short, and it should be based on the things that are most likely to derail your diet, exercise, or lifestyle.

KEEP YOUR LIST PRIVATE, BUT KEEP IT CLOSE BY

You are not going to show your list to your family.

In fact, you're not even going to mention that you came up with a list of areas you need help in. As I'll explain in the next chapter, this list is for your own clarity, so that you can better explain to your family the areas you're struggling with, and they can then help you come up with solutions.

Part of the reason for writing this list down, however, is so that you can remind yourself of the things that you need help with. Using this list as a reminder will keep you focused, but it will also make you much more appreciative when your family starts helping you in the ways that you need.

Only by taking this approach will you be able to invest your family in your success, which is crucial if you want to get their full support and encouragement. You must have some idea of how your family can help you first. Once you do, it's time to have a conversation with them.

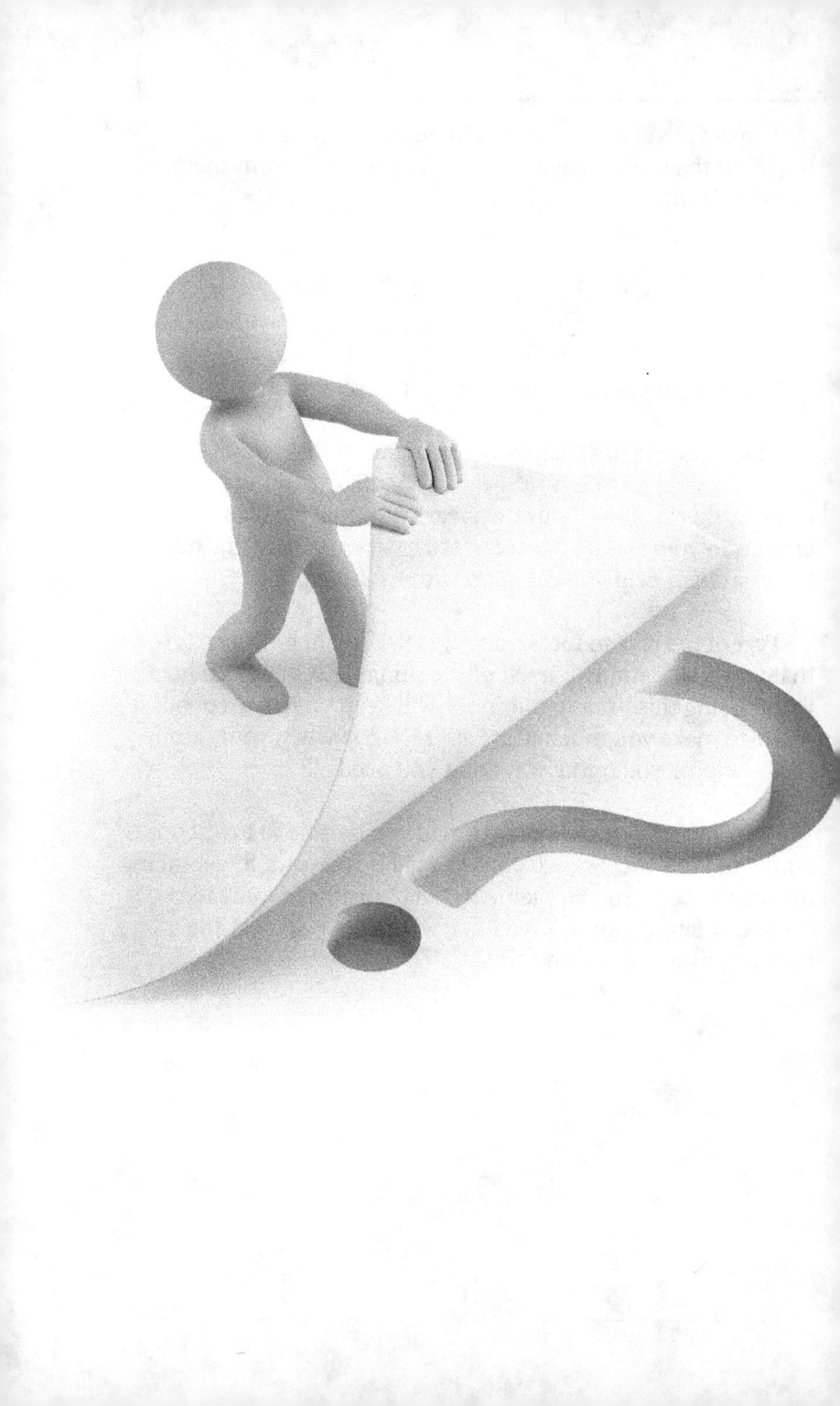

CHAPTER 4:
HOW TO ASK YOUR FAMILY FOR SUPPORT AND ENCOURAGEMENT

Once you know which areas you really need help with in your diet or health plan, it's time to start involving your family. Up until now, everything has been about changing your own mindset and getting clear on what it is you really need to ask for help with. At this point, though, everything suddenly changes and is about your family.

And having these conversations is the hardest part, by far. When we talk to our spouse/partner or our kids, we often fall into old habits and routines. Quite often, our conversations with them are not very open or interactive.

This is not your fault or their fault, but you need to be the one who takes responsibility for changing it.

In this chapter, I'm going to focus on starting conversations that recruit your family to help you eat better and live a better lifestyle. However, learning to have better and more open conversations with your family (or with anybody) will reverberate throughout your life.

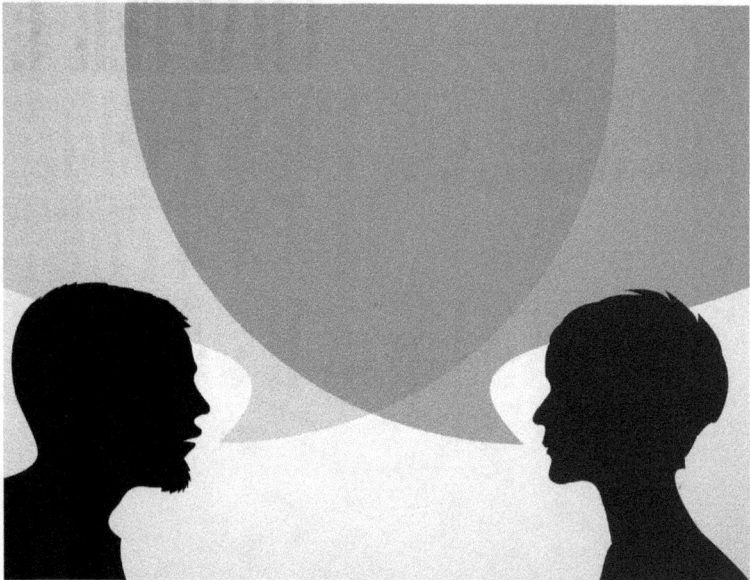

THE "CAN YOU HELP ME WIN?" CONVERSATION

The conversation that you need to have with each member of your immediate family is something I call the "Can You Help Me Win?" conversation.

I like this name for two reasons.

First, **this conversation is a question, and that's how you have to approach it**. You can't go in assuming that they can or will help you. They might even say no the first few times you ask. However, if you approach it already knowing that they can and should help you, then you are simply trying to force them to help, rather than giving them the opportunity to play an important role.

Second, although I don't think you always need to think about health, dieting, and nutrition as something you can "win," it helps in this case, because **you want to get your family invested in and excited about your success.** You're going to give them an opportunity to be the heroes who help carry you across the finish line. If you can build that kind of excitement and enthusiasm, and if you can give them the chance to play a big role, then everything will be easy.

Below is a step-by-step process to having this conversation, but let me make one thing clear.

Have this conversation one person at a time.

We all have pictures in our mind of various television shows where the entire family sits down (to dinner or otherwise) and has a big family conversation about an important topic. In those ideal TV situations, there might be a little bit of struggle, but it very quickly ends with the whole family hugging and crying tears of joy. That's not usually how it goes in real life. It's possible, but it's much more likely that you'll be successful if you deal with each member of your family one at a time.

HOW TO HAVE THE CONVERSATION

You can't read a script for a conversation. If you did, it wouldn't be a conversation at all.

And this conversation is NOT going to feel comfortable. But it gets easier over time.

Fortunately, although you can't read a script, you can follow a basic outline. This outline is something that I've used many times in my own life, and it's something that I know others have had success with. Just remember that it's a guide, and no conversation you ever have will go exactly according to plan. That's OK, and even if you mess it up the first 99 times, if you get it right on the 100th try, then you're probably going to end up with the support and encouragement that you're looking for.

As an aside, I also want to say that nothing in this outline is meant to trick anybody you're talking to in any way. In a few cases, I mention that approaching the conversation in a certain way will make your spouse/partner or child more likely to respond favorably. Really, what they're going to respond most favorably to is a genuine request for help, and this outline is simply a way to facilitate you doing that.

1. Ask if they have time to talk.

In order to start the conversation off on the right foot, your spouse/partner or child needs to actually agree to have a conversation (especially tough sometimes when it comes to teenagers). You don't have to ask this in a particularly serious way. You could ask "Do you have a minute?" or "Can I ask you about something?"

Always make it a question, because you need to get an affirmative reply. Once you've gotten one affirmative reply, they're much more likely to engage and listen.

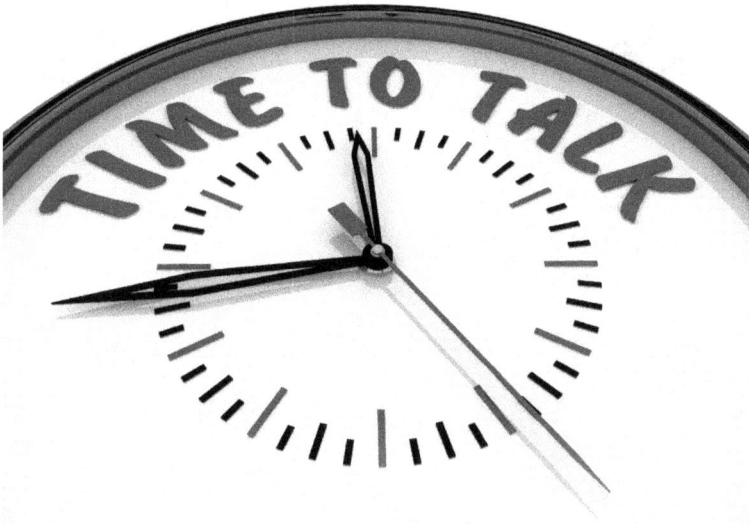

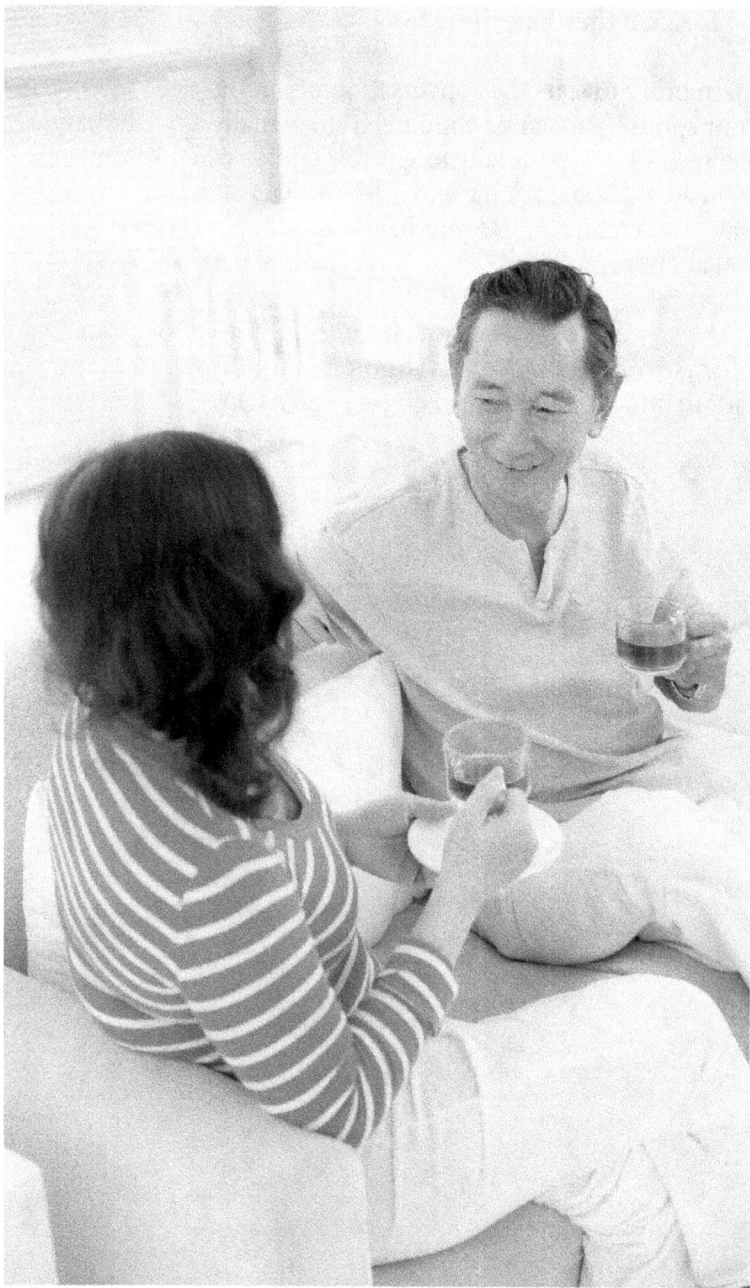

2. Tell them why you want to have this conversation.

This should be brief, but it should include three things: (a) your goal, (b) why that goal is important to you, and (c) that you want them to help you.

Say these things in a very positive way. Fake it if you have to. For instance, maybe you're interested in losing 20 pounds of fat. If so, then the conversation should start with a simple statement of what you'd like (losing 20 lbs) and why that's important to you (want to look better, scared of developing disease, more energy, etc.). For example, you could say, "I would like to lose 20 lbs in the next 3 months so that I can start feeling better every day. It'd really improve my health."

Do NOT use this as a time to complain. Don't start listing out all of your complaints about how fat you've gotten or how bad you've felt. It's ok to feel that way, but you want to use this conversation as an opportunity to get your spouse/partner or kids excited about a better future. Focusing on present or past problems will quickly turn the conversation toward a negative point of view.

3. Point out why they are uniquely qualified to help.

Maybe it's just because they live with you or because they're the person you spend the most time with. However, try to come up with a couple genuine reasons why they'll be particularly good at helping you achieve your goals.

Are they always positive and encouraging? Have they achieved big goals in their own life, even if it was a long time ago? If they're stubborn, maybe that's a sign of grit and determination?

Honestly, step back and think about how their qualities are a great fit to help you reach your own goals, whether it's weight loss, feeling better, exercising more, eating healthier, or anything else. And let them know that you recognize their strengths.

(The primary purpose of doing this might seem like it's just to make them feel good, and that's certainly one purpose. But this step also helps you really appreciate what they bring to the table, which makes it much more likely that you're approaching this conversation with a good and positive mindset.)

So, you might say something like this: "I've always found your dedication and perseverance working your own way through college really inspiring, and I think getting your support would really help me to build those same qualities too and help me stick to my health plan."

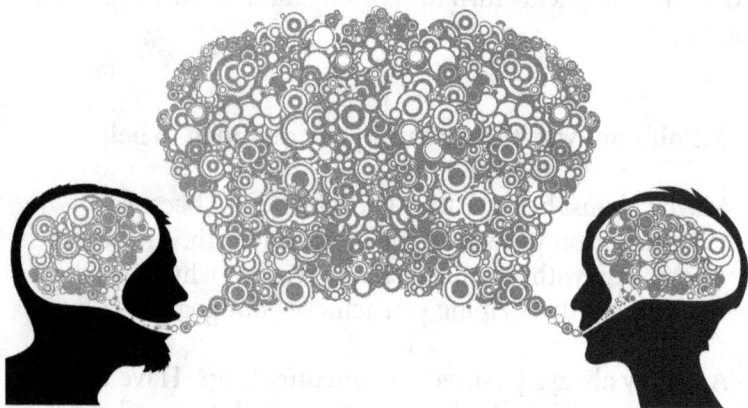

4.   Ask them if they might be willing to help you reach your goal and if they have any thoughts.

This is really important. You've opened up the conversation by asking if they have time to chat, very quickly laying out what you're thinking, and then telling them why you think they could help a lot. If you haven't already gotten them talking, then you need to start asking more questions at this point. Perhaps just something simple like, "What do you think?"

Ask for their opinion, their feedback, any concerns they have, and any extra ideas that they might have for helping you.

During this part of the conversation, really acknowledge their suggestions and thoughts. Repeat back to them what they're saying, as it will acknowledge that you hear them. You don't have to agree with everything they say in order to understand that they're already trying to help.

Do NOT immediately launch into how you plan to accomplish your goal. I know that you already have a plan in your mind, but try as hard as you can to make this a conversation whereby you actually listen to their suggestions and thoughts. And don't expect all of their suggestions/thoughts to fit in with what you've been thinking.

Your spouse/kids might start out by trying to convince you that you don't need to do this – that you don't need to eat better or lose weight. Most of the time, that's just their way of trying to make you feel better. If they're doing this, then that is a GREAT SIGN. In other words, they hear how you feel and want to make you feel better. They're just not yet helping you in the way that you believe will make the most difference. **But they clearly care.**

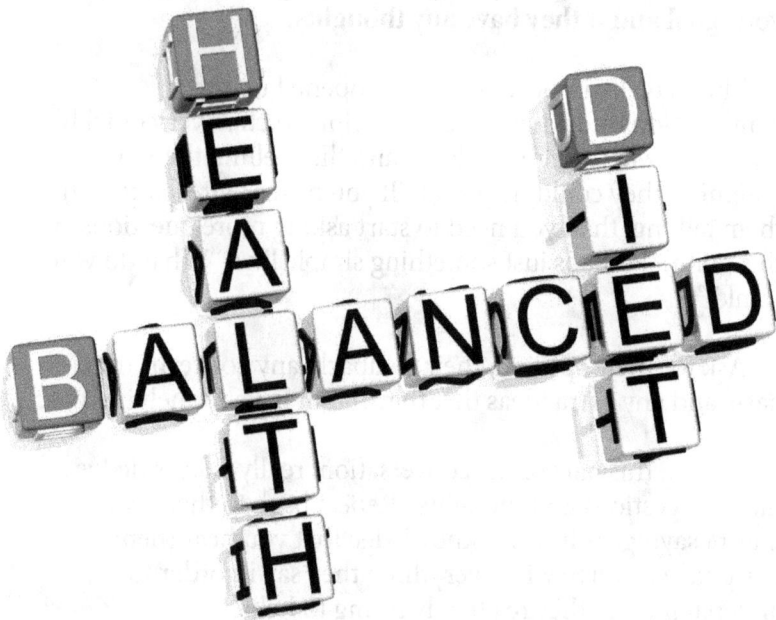

5.   Ask your spouse/partner or your kids about specific ideas they have to help you reach your specific goals.

This step is really just an extension of step #4, but after you've opened up the discussion, you should definitely mention the general approach to reaching your specific goals that you've been thinking about.

For instance, let's say that you've decided to try to lose 20 pounds by going on a particular diet. You should not try convincing your family that your chosen diet or approach is the right solution to your problems. Your spouse/partner or kids don't really care what the right solution is. But they do care that you're happy and able to achieve the goals that are important to you.

In Chapter 3, you came up with a short list of ways that your spouse/partner or kids can potentially help you stick to your diet/lifestyle. For this part of the conversation, you should have those ways in mind, but don't jump right out and say "I've come up with a list of ways that I want you to help me. #1…."

If you take that approach, then their immediate reaction is going to be that you're just trying to force them to do something for your own benefit, that everything is your idea, and that they really have very little value.

So your conversation here might be just: "I've been hearing a lot about a diet that my friend used to lose weight, and it seems to be about healing and nourishing my body with healthy foods rather than just depriving me of food. I'd love to know whether you think I could benefit from trying something like that."

6. Be willing to adapt the ways they can help you.

This is the tough part of the conversation. On one hand, you don't want to come unprepared with no idea of how your family member can help you out. If you do that, then the conversation is most likely to end in a vague way, with your spouse or child saying that they'll definitely help you out, but without any particular plan for how they'll help you. On the other hand, if you try to force your imagined ways of them helping you, then they'll feel like they weren't a part of the process and therefore will be uncommitted to your goals.

What needs to happen is that you need to tell them the areas that you see as a potential problem for you, then be willing to adapt the plan based on their feedback. Here is a good example.

Imagine that a big problem for you is that your spouse always brings home junk food (cookies and crackers), and then you have a very hard time not eating the junk when it's around the house. This is a very common occurrence.

When you came up with your list of ways that your spouse could potentially help you, you might have written down "don't buy or bring home any cookies or crackers." And for you, that would probably go a long way toward helping you stick to your diet.

During your conversation with your spouse, you might mention that one big area of concern for you is that you have a hard time not eating junk food like cookies and crackers that you see around the house. And then you'd ask your spouse if there was any way that they might be able to help you out with that concern.

Their response might be, "OK, how about this – I'll lock all of the junk food in my home office, and I won't eat any of it in front of you."

Their response is probably not your ideal solution, but it's not a bad one. If your spouse's home office is a room that you never go into, and if they never eat the junk food when you're around, then you'll probably be much less tempted.

The point here is that you can't go into the conversation expecting to get exactly the outcome that you want. The outcome you should really be aiming for is to simply get some commitments from your spouse and kids to help you stick to your diet/lifestyle and succeed at your goals. If you get that outcome, then everything else will eventually fall into place.

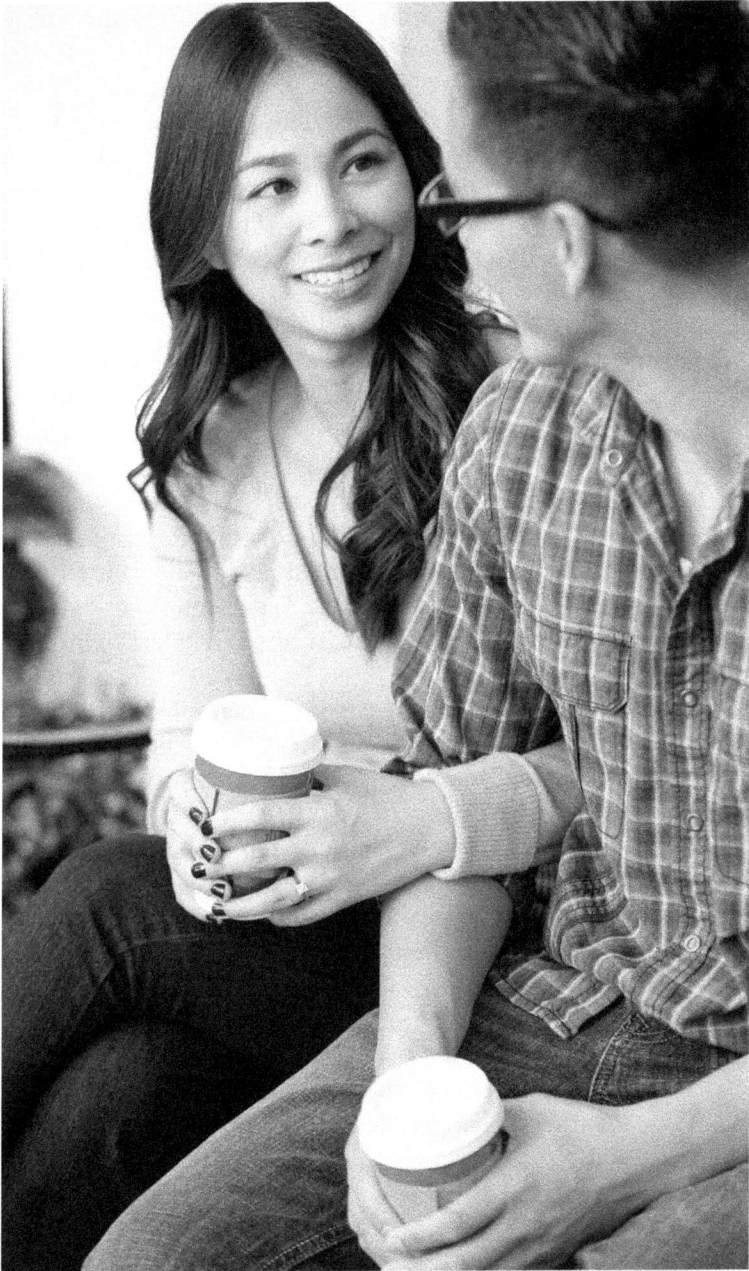

7.   Set an expectation for future conversations and for check-ins.

Once you've started this conversation, you most certainly don't want to end it too soon (or ever). Toward the end of the conversation, tell them how much you've appreciated discussing this with them (even if it hasn't been 100% pleasant), and ask if they're willing to discuss it again with you in a few days or a week to see how you're doing, to check in on your progress, and to figure out if there are any other ways that they can help you.

I like to suggest periodic check-ins (either daily or weekly) where your spouse or kids ask you how you're doing with whatever it is you're trying to accomplish. This serves 2 purposes. First, it provides an easy opportunity for more conversations later, and second, it mentally invests your family in your success. It's hard for someone to continually ask you how you're doing and not start to care about it at least a little.

One bit of caution about the periodic check-ins. Remember that your spouse or kids are asking you how you're doing because you wanted them to care. That means if you're having a bad day (maybe you had a cookie at work or didn't sleep well the night before), you should remember not to take it out on them. Try not to snap back with "Don't ask!" or "Stop getting on my case," because it'll send the message to them that you don't want them to ask EVER.

ACTION STEP #3:
Use the Framework Above to Have Your First
"Can You Help Me Win?" Conversation.

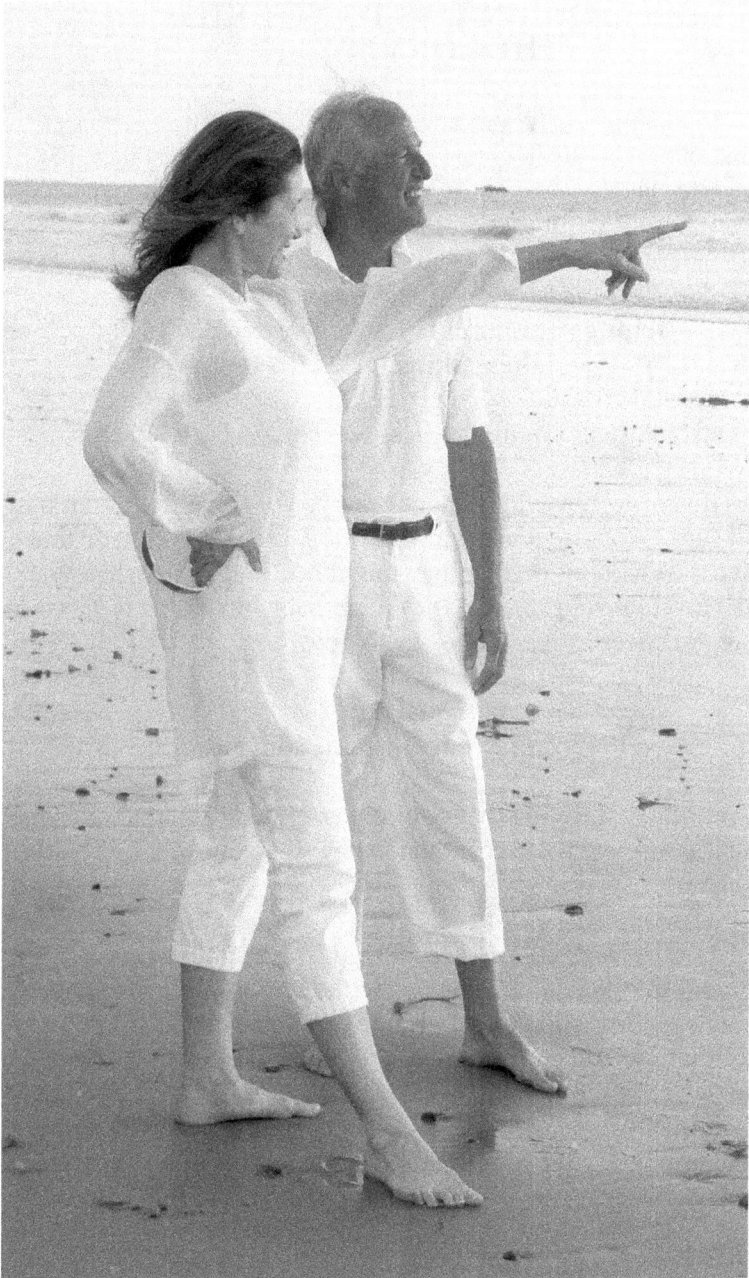

QUICK TIPS TO NOT KILL
THE CONVERSATION

In Chapter 8, I've got a whole list of common mistakes that people make in general, but here are a few mistakes that people specifically make when having a conversation with their family about diet, health, and nutrition:

Mistake #1:
Telling your family what you've decided to do,
and then asking for their support.

It's got to be a mutual process. Period.

If you start by telling them what you're going to do (cut out all sugar, exercise 5 times a week, etc.), then you've made that decision without them. They might nod and smile when you ask for their support, but they're probably not going to be your biggest cheerleaders a week from now.

Mistake #2:
Planning to have just one conversation.

If you're thinking that one conversation is going to get you all the support you need, then you're still viewing it as a battle with your family.

In other words, you're thinking of your spouse/partner or children as people to be converted or else conquered in a single battle. And you're certainly not thinking of this as a mutual and interactive process.

When you view this as a golden opportunity to improve and enhance your relationship with your family, you'll actually want to have future conversations with them about this topic, because each conversation will serve to make your relationship that much better.

Plus, there's no guarantee that the first conversation is going to go well. Many of my conversations with Louise still don't go well. But as time goes on, they tend to get better and better.

Mistake #3:
Not showing appreciation.

You MUST do this. And you should do it all the time.

First of all, before they even start helping you, show appreciation during your conversations with your family for the skills and talents that they have that might help you to succeed. Maybe they're creative or very organized – all qualities that can be helpful for someone trying to change their diet and lifestyle.

And then once your family starts supporting and encouraging you, find little ways to continually thank them.

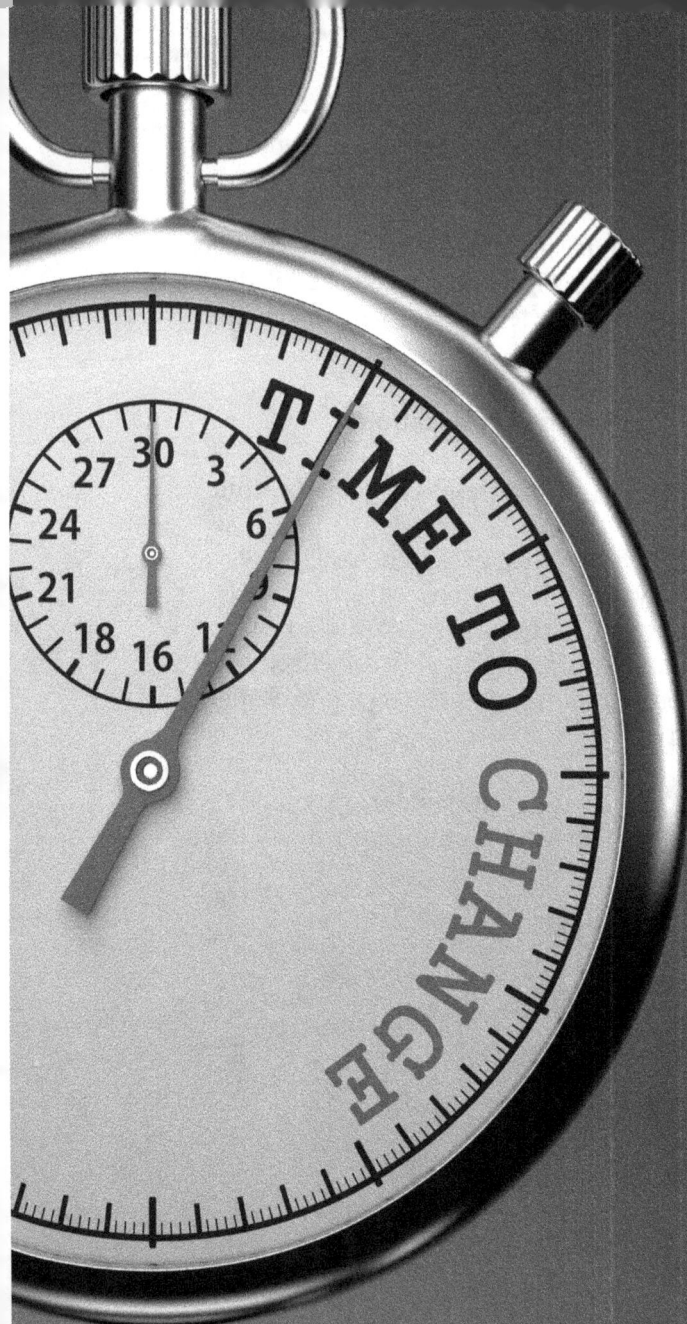

CHAPTER 5:
HOW TO CONVERT YOUR FAMILY TO A HEALTHIER WAY OF EATING AND LIVING

Both Louise's and my parents have a number of health problems, from heart conditions to diabetes to a variety of undiagnosed ailments. So we have a strong inclination to help them get healthier.

Consequently, Louise and I have spent most of the past 5 years trying to convince our parents to eat better and live a healthier lifestyle.

And remember our situation - Louise and I have been studying health and nutrition with the best doctors and scientists in the world for around a decade. We publish 2 popular health magazines and write blogs that have thousands of readers per day. On a personal level, I've lost a ton of weight, and Louise has cured several illnesses that her doctors had no answer for.

And yet...our parents still doubt or resist every single change that we encourage.

It took me many years to develop my Super-Secret and Simple System for Changing Your Family's Health and Diet. Here it is:

DON'T TRY.

You should never try to convert any member of your family to your way of thinking about diet, health, or nutrition. The only exception to this rule is a young child, and that's something I discuss in the next chapter.

MOST OF US MAKE IT LESS LIKELY THAT OUR FAMILY WILL CHANGE

If you are actively trying to convert your family to your way of thinking about diet, nutrition, or health, then 2 things will happen:

1.   You will get tired and burnt out, and you will give up.
2.   You will make it less likely that they'll change than if you hadn't tried to convert them.

There are certainly exceptions, but that has been the experience of nearly everyone I've spoken with or helped on this issue. And there is a reason why this is the case.

The very act of trying to convert a family member (or even a friend) implicitly means that you view their behavior or beliefs as wrong or bad in some way. You probably aren't consciously thinking that they are wrong, but then again, you wouldn't be trying to get them to change if you didn't think that there was a better way for them to live, eat, or think.

To be fair, you might be right. Maybe their diet or lifestyle is very unhealthy for them, and they're just thinking about it in a bad way. But nobody wants to believe that they're wrong.

So what happens is that the person you're trying to change will get defensive. And when that happens, they will start to justify what they're doing – both to you and to themselves. And ironically, that very act of justification strengthens their resolve to stick to their way of eating or living.

For example, if you try to convince your spouse that they're doing a lot of damage to their body by eating junk food all the time, then you're probably correct. However, their reaction is likely to be defensive, and they might justify themselves and their way of eating by saying that they would prefer to eat yummy food rather than be healthy and deprive themselves or that they'd rather eat their delicious junk foods and die early than suffer a lifetime of eating your "healthy" foods.

Before you tried to convince your spouse, they might not have even been thinking about why they ate junk food, and they probably didn't even have a good reason. But once you start trying to convince them that they're wrong to eat those foods, they quickly develop a personal identity (as someone who values food over health). Once that happens, it becomes much less likely that they're going to change.

I know this from both first- and second-hand experiences. Louise's dad really has no objection to eating healthier, but when we try to pressure him to do it, he immediately tells us that life's not worth living if he can't just eat whatever he wants. I don't think he truly believes this, but it's easier to justify his actions this way than to admit that he's choosing to eat in a way that hurts himself.

Louise and I hate seeing any of our family or friends eat food or live a lifestyle that we know is bad for them and will cause them a lot of pain or health problems. And in those cases, it's hard to sit by and not try to convince them that what they're doing is harmful.

And yet, it's the most effective way.

3 SIMPLE RULES FOR HELPING FAMILY AND FRIENDS

There is no guide or step-by-step system for converting your family – or anybody else for that matter.

But there are 3 simple rules that will put you in a great position should any family member or friend be ready to make a change:

1. Live as Healthy as You Can. Stick to your guns, and be a beacon. But don't do it for that reason. Do it because you want to be healthy and you know that eating well and living a healthy lifestyle makes everything in your own life better.

2. Ask for the Help of Others. Be sensitive to what your family and friends want, but never feel like your diet or your health are a burden to them. Instead, view your diet and lifestyle as a golden opportunity to let them share in and contribute to your success.

3. Help When Asked. If a family member or friend does come to you for help or advice about health, diet, or nutrition, then ask them how you can best help them. It may not be the way that you think is best, but unless you think it's going to harm them (like taking dangerous pills or starving themselves), then give them your full support.

Again, these 3 rules will put you in a position to help should your spouse, kids, or anybody else be ready to ask you for help, but it's not a plan to convert your family or friends. That choice is theirs, and if you truly want them to support you in your choices, you will need to do the same for them.

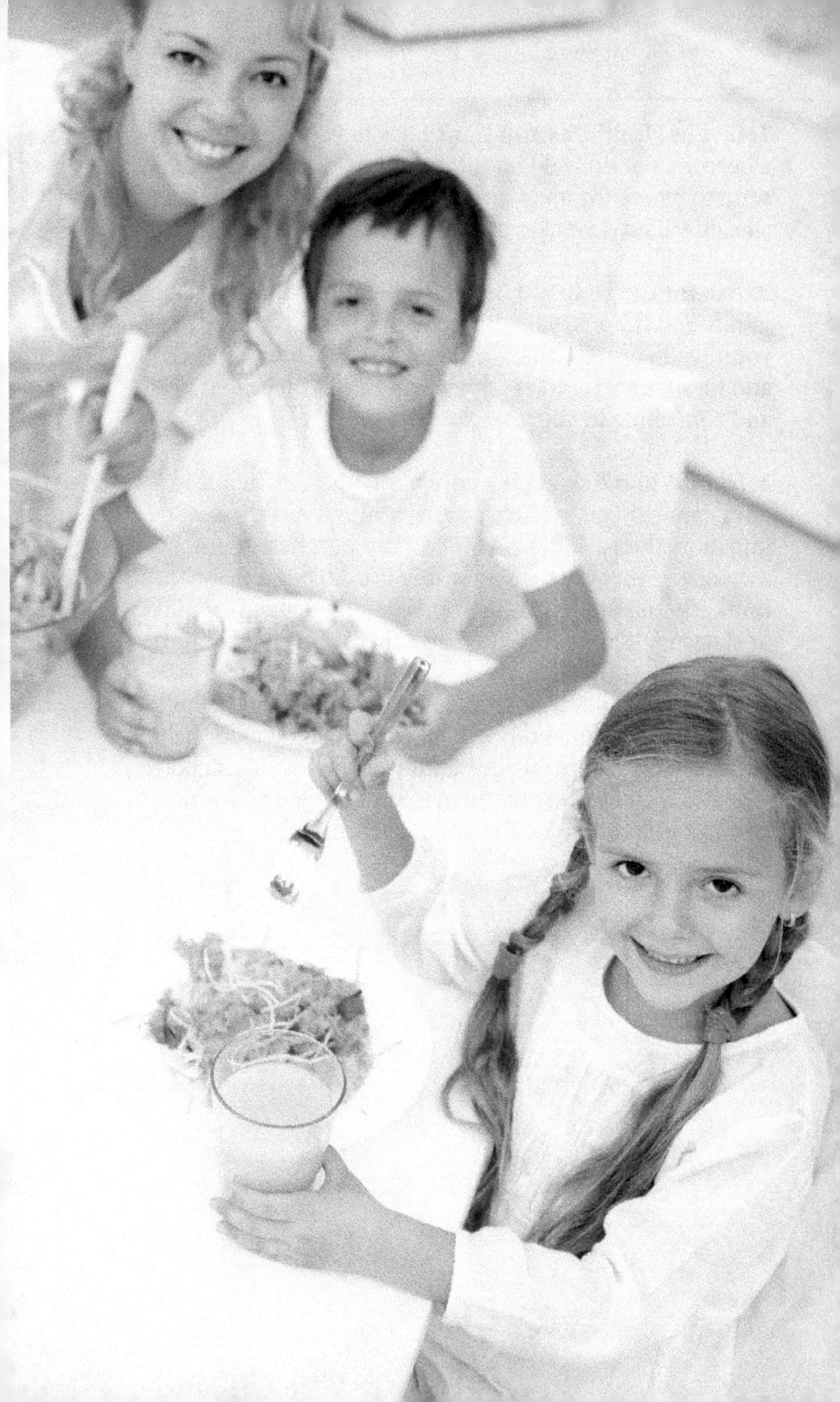

CHAPTER 6:
HOW TO GAIN THE SUPPORT OF YOUNG CHILDREN

You might think, in theory, that a young child is easier to convince or change.

In actuality, you'd only *occasionally* be right.

For the most part, I've written this book because so many people told me about the trouble they were having sticking to their diets while their spouse, partner, or older children were making different choices. In each case, you need to involve them, make them feel like a valuable and meaningful part of your success, and have ongoing discussions that show them your appreciation for helping you.

If you have young children, though, then it's a completely different matter. (I generally consider a child "young" in this respect until he or she is about 7 or 8.) It can still be a situation that makes it harder for you, but I believe that you need to approach this situation just a little bit differently compared to other members of your family.

YOUNG CHILDREN WANT TO HELP YOU EVEN MORE

It's true. Even the most rebellious child really wants to please you.

They might not show it in the way you like, but if you can harness that desire to help and please you, then they'll be your biggest supporters.

So even more than your spouse, partner, or older kids, you need to enlist the support of young kids. If you tell them that you're trying to eat better so that you'll feel good yourself, young children will often jump at the chance to help. (They might forget often – they're kids after all – but it's easy to remind them how they wanted to help you out.)

Use every opportunity you can to get their help, and then show them how much you appreciate even the little things they do to help you eat and feel better.

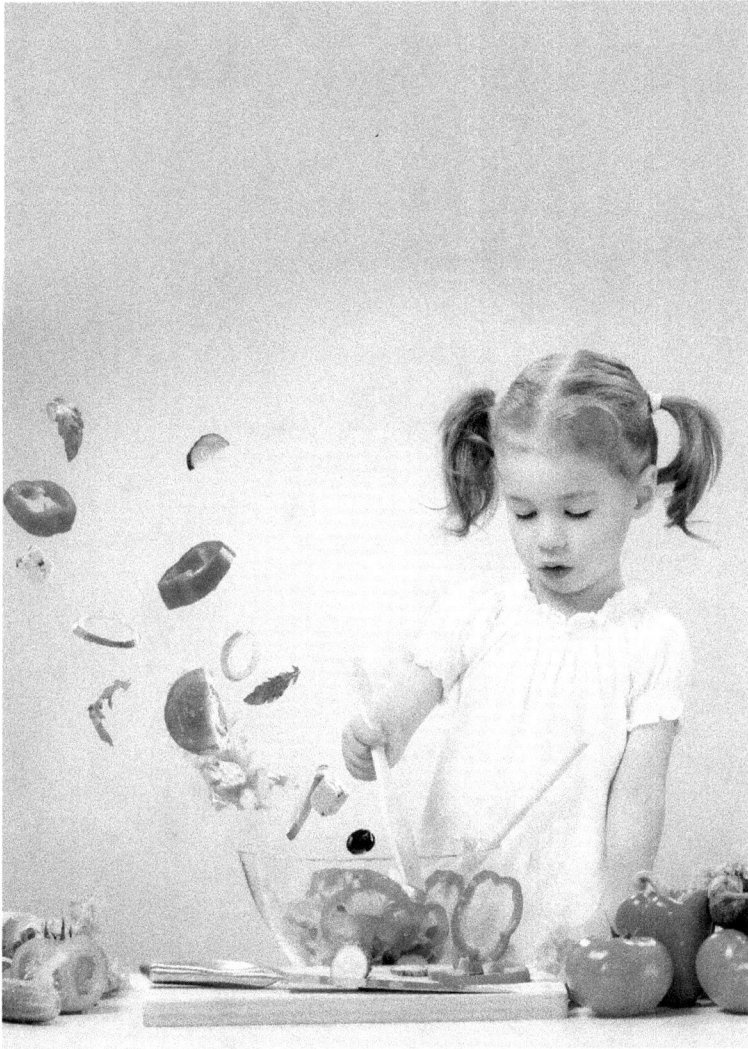

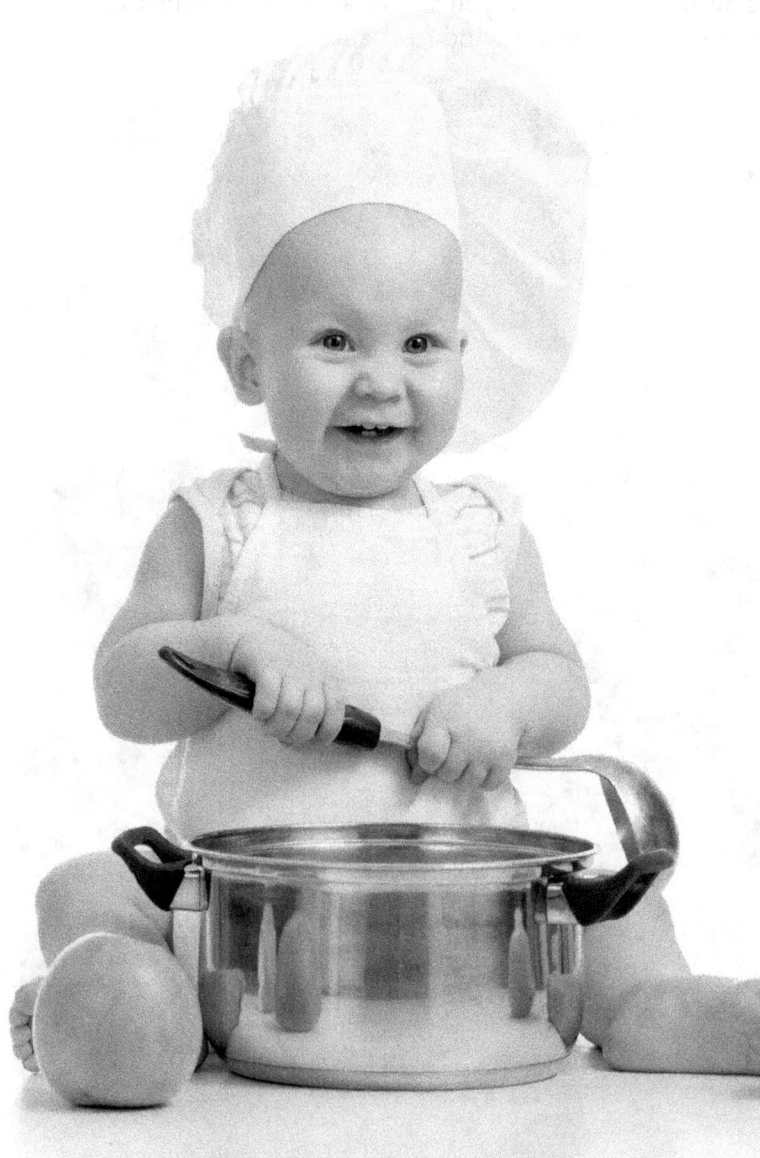

YOU NEED TO EDUCATE YOUNG CHILDREN

This is a big difference from your older kids or your spouse or partner. Even if you believe that they don't understand something, your job is not to educate them.

On the other hand, young kids need to learn. But they don't just need to learn facts. **They need to learn how to make good and healthy decisions about their food and their bodies.** Unlike you and me, they often don't yet recognize the roles that food, exercise, and lifestyle have on their bodies.

And there are a lot of good ways that you can get them to start thinking about it.

Involve them in cooking and food preparation. The parents who are most successful at getting their kids interested in health and nutrition are those who involve them in the preparation and cooking of meals at a very early age. It stands to reason that if a child feels like they play an important role in preparing food, then they also feel responsible for choosing and preparing food that makes everybody feel good (once they understand how that works).

Talk to them about how they feel. Ask them if they think a food will make them feel good or feel bad. And when they do feel bad after eating something (like too much candy), have an honest discussion with them about what made them feel bad. The point is not to scare them away from junk food or candy but to get them to start independently thinking about how foods affect their bodies. This is something that very young children can easily understand.

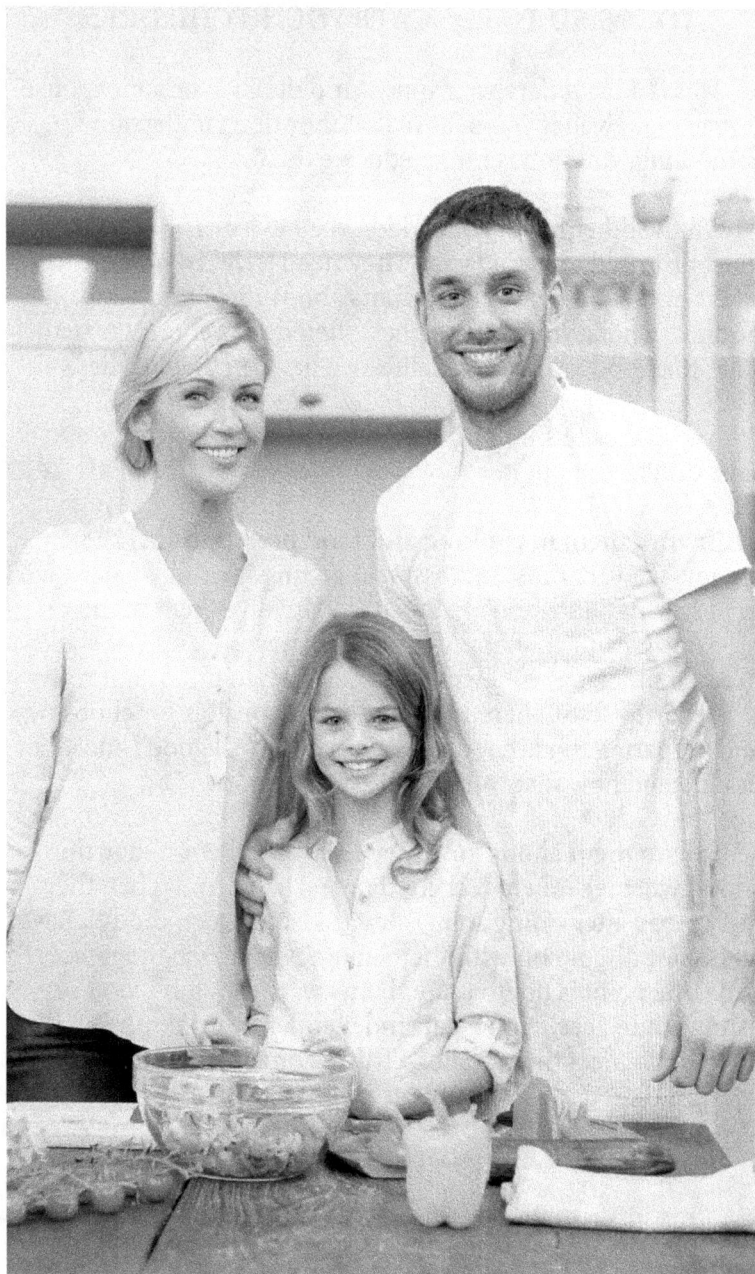

YOUNG CHILDREN SHOULDN'T MAKE ALL OF THEIR OWN FOOD CHOICES

Here are 2 things that I'm **not** saying: (a) that you should try to brainwash your children into thinking about diet and nutrition just like you; or (b) that you shouldn't involve them at all in the decision-making process.

However, young kids should not be given the choice of eating junk just because they don't yet understand what it does to them. If you can afford to buy and feed them high quality and nutritious food, then it's your responsibility to do so, even if they yell and scream about it.

By all means, have conversations with your 4- or 5-year-old to get them more interested in health and nutrition, so that they'll eventually make the best decisions. Just don't use their current thoughts or temper tantrums as an excuse to feed them junk. You're not doing them any favors.

TREAT THEM LIKE ADULTS

In every other way, you should really treat them like adults. Have ongoing conversations with them to try to get their support for eating better and living a healthier lifestyle. Come up with specific ways that they can help you, and also encourage them to think of some ways.

When they see that they're actually helping you and that you value their opinion and help, they'll also be the first people to voluntarily change their own way of eating. And in the end, that will make your life a whole lot easier.

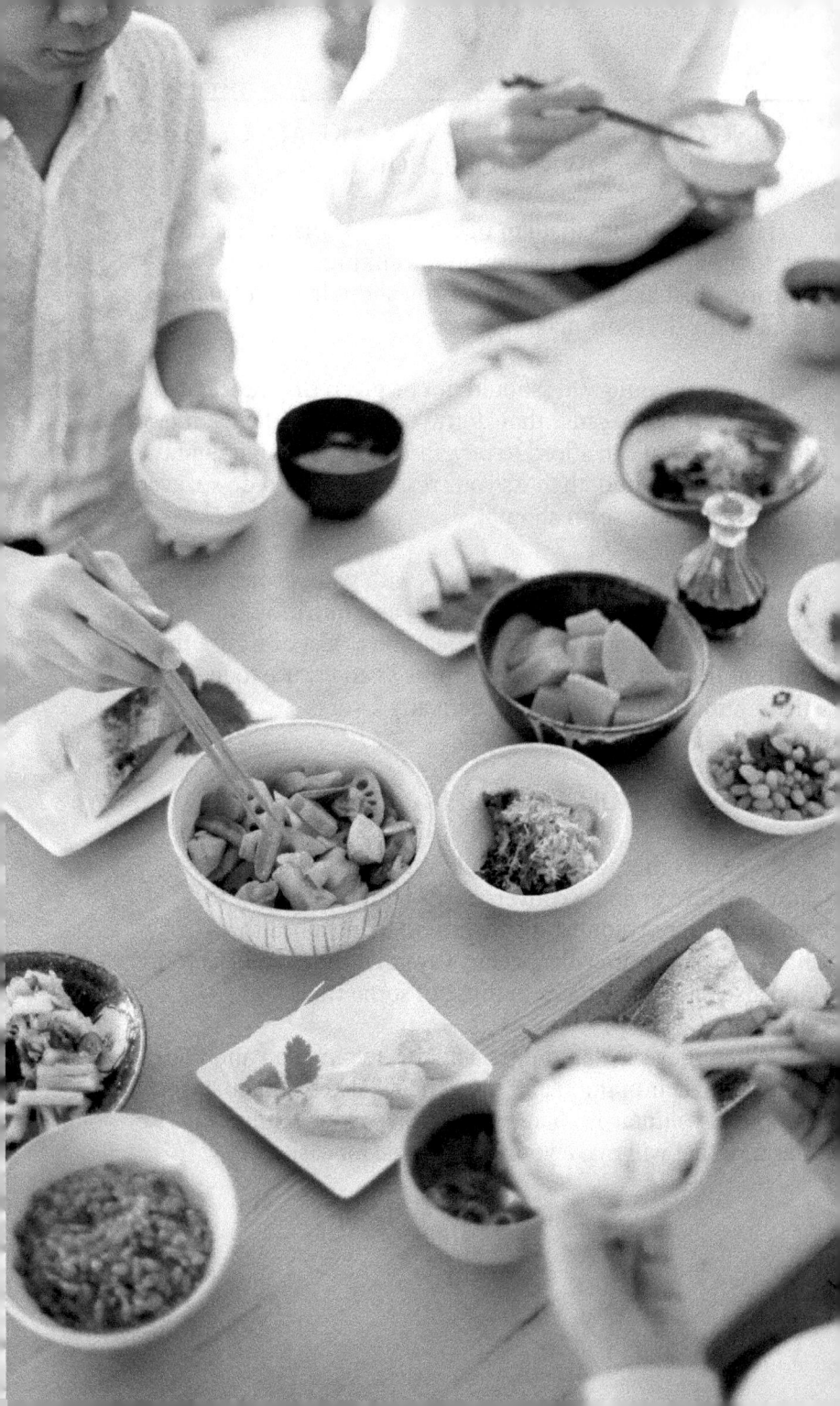

CHAPTER 7: FRIENDS AND EXTENDED FAMILY

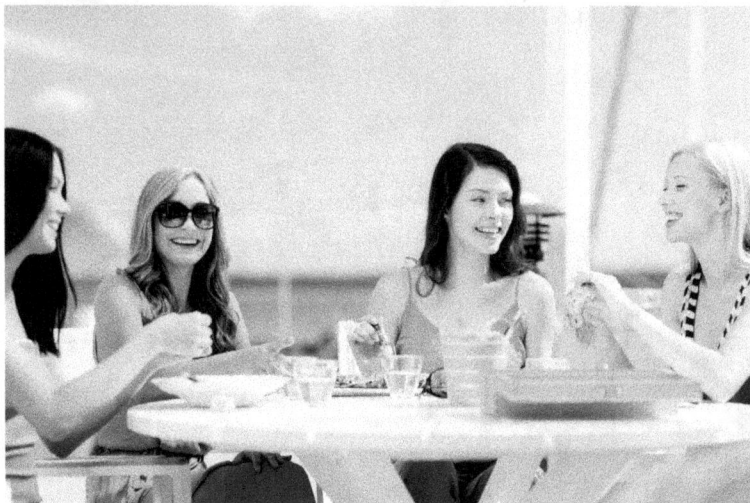

I have written this book to help you gain the support, encouragement, and eventually, the participation of your spouse or partner, and also your children.

My focus is on your immediate family because, 95% of the time, those are the people with whom you live and who are most important to your success or failure at maintaining a healthy diet and lifestyle.

And ironically, these are often the hardest people to deal with. Our interactions with our immediate family are often ruled by habits and rituals, so having new and different conversations with them is usually tough, especially if our kids are older or if we've been with our spouse/partner for a very long time.

Nonetheless, the techniques in this book are applicable to any family member and even to close friends.

When you approach your friends, you need to have the

same mentality, that your diet is a golden opportunity to let them help you. But even more so than your immediate family, you need to have in mind a very short list of ways that they can help you.

Your friends also want to support and encourage you, but they're not always around, so the ways that they can help you out are different. And you need to keep that in mind when you have conversations with them.

The point is, if there is somebody in your life whose support your need for your diet/lifestyle changes, then the approach that I've outlined in this book will work for you.

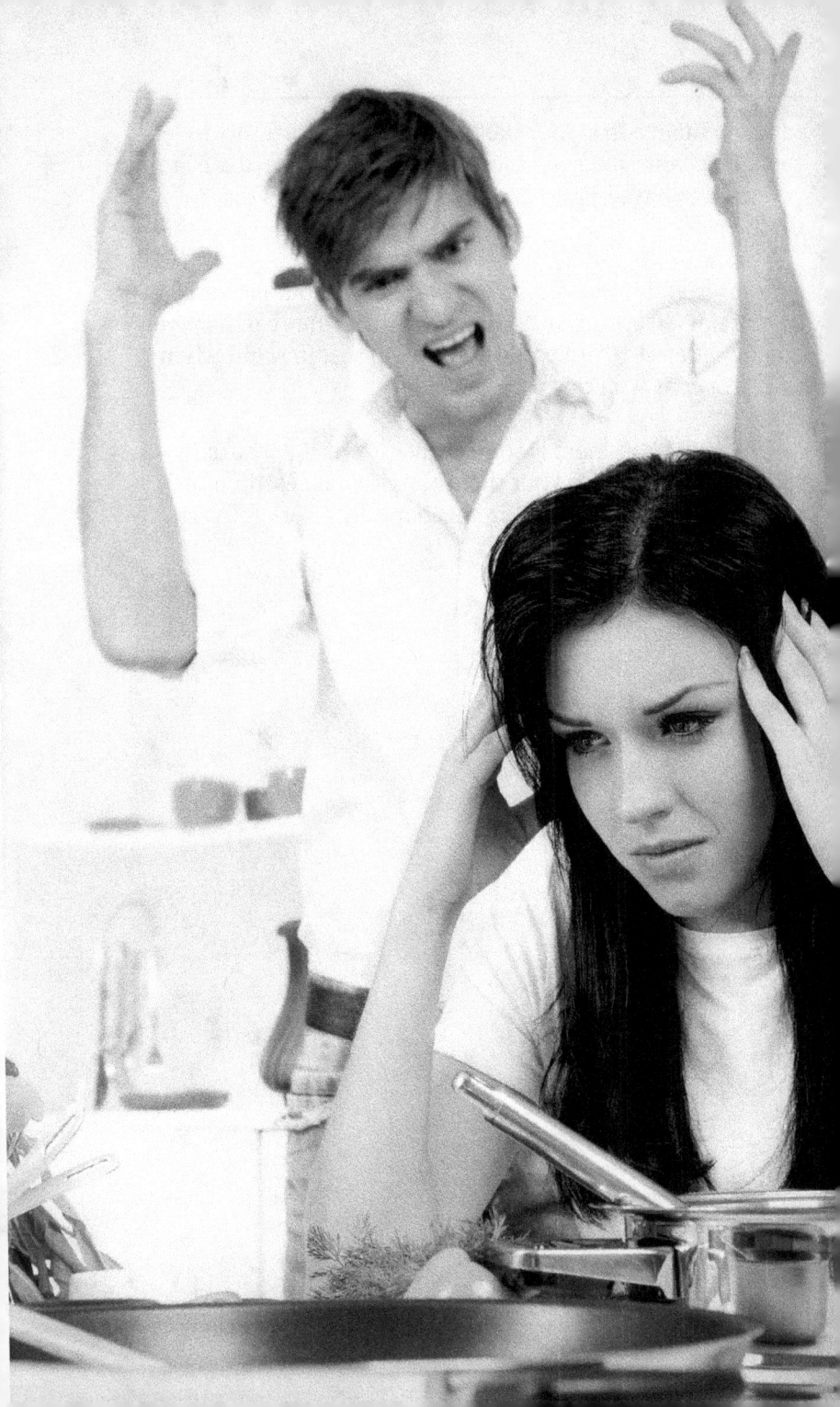

CHAPTER 8:
COMMON MISTAKES THAT DOOM FOLKS

There are a lot of reasons why we don't have perfect relationships, and there are a lot of reasons why it's hard to change your diet, to exercise more or better, and to just get healthier.

But after talking to thousands of people about this, I tend to see 4 common mistakes creep up over and over again.

MISTAKE #1: Trying to Convert Your Family. I see a lot of people succeed in moving their family to healthy, real-food diets. But I see very few people do it by trying to convert their families.

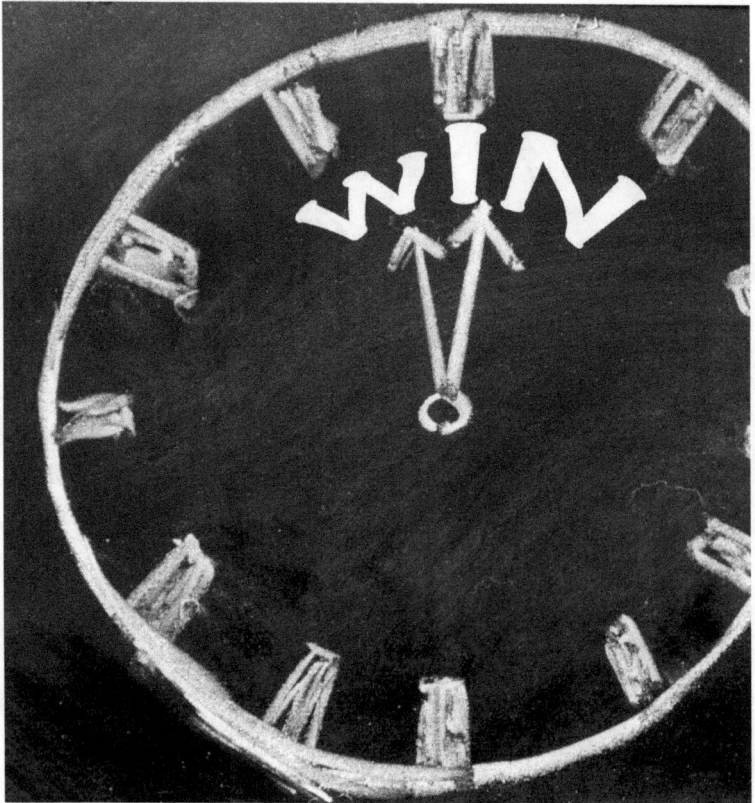

In Chapter 5, I talked about this in a lot of detail, but the takeaway in the end is that you're much better off (and more likely to convert your family) if you simply get them to support you.

MISTAKE #2: Believing Your Partner, Spouse, or Child is "Stubborn." I hear this continually. Women in particular tell me that their husband or boyfriend is too stubborn to change or to help them out.

I'm going to refrain from opining on whether or not men are more stubborn. It doesn't matter. No matter who it is, this is a bad mindset to start with, because you're going to approach them already believing that you'll fail.

And the reason you'll fail is not because they're stubborn, but rather because you were trying to change their mind or their opinion. The better way is to tap into what you already have (that they care about you), and use the tactics from Chapters 2 and 3 to get them to support you.

MISTAKE #3: Never Giving Your Family Their Golden Opportunity. The entire reason I wrote this book is because I believe that so many people are missing out on this golden opportunity to deepen their relationships with their family. And for me, so much of the reason to improve our bodies and our health is based on creating and enjoying better relationships.

I know that many people who read this book will never take any of the actions that I know have worked for many, many people. And that's OK. But if you're reading this right now, don't be one of those people. Give both yourself and your family the opportunity to help you succeed, get healthier, and improve your time together.

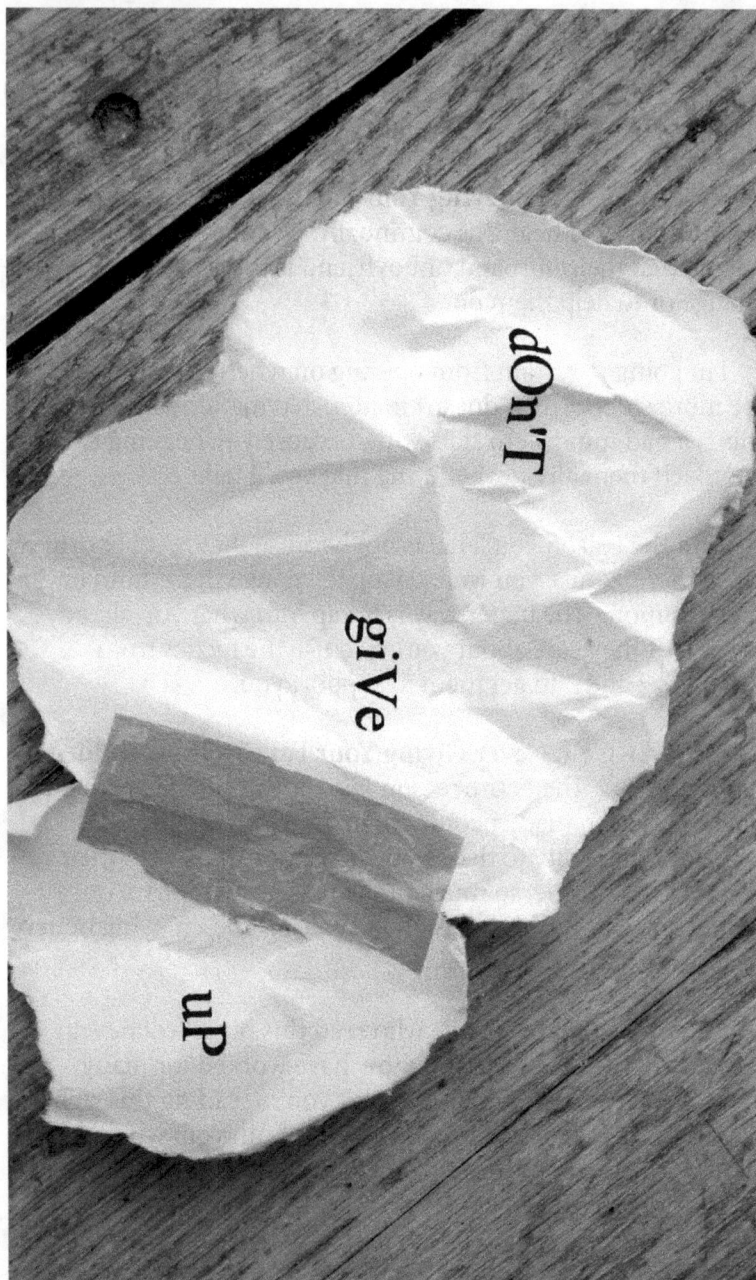

MISTAKE #4: Giving Up. This is the most unfortunate mistake, but it's the one I can relate to the most. I often want to give up when things aren't going well, and sometimes relationships are going to take work.

That includes how you and your family deal with food, exercise, sleep, and other aspects of your health. You'll have good conversations and they'll support you and cheer you on, but you'll also have times when you feel like nothing is going right and nobody is helping you out.

Often, that's simply because you're looking at the situation as a problem and picking out all of the things that are going wrong, when, in actuality, many more things are going right. I catch myself doing this all the time.

Even if you have weeks at a time that are not great, don't give up, either on your health or on the chance to use your health to improve your relationships. I promise that the time and effort will pay off in the end.

MISTAKE #5: Not Doing the Work. I would love to have you read this book and magically improve everything about your health, diet, family, and relationships. But if all you do is read this book and then put it away, you'll get very little out of it.

You're going to need to do some work – particularly on the way that you think about your diet and health – and you're also going to need to do some work on how you communicate with your family.

There's a helpful Cheat Sheet at the end of this book - USE IT!

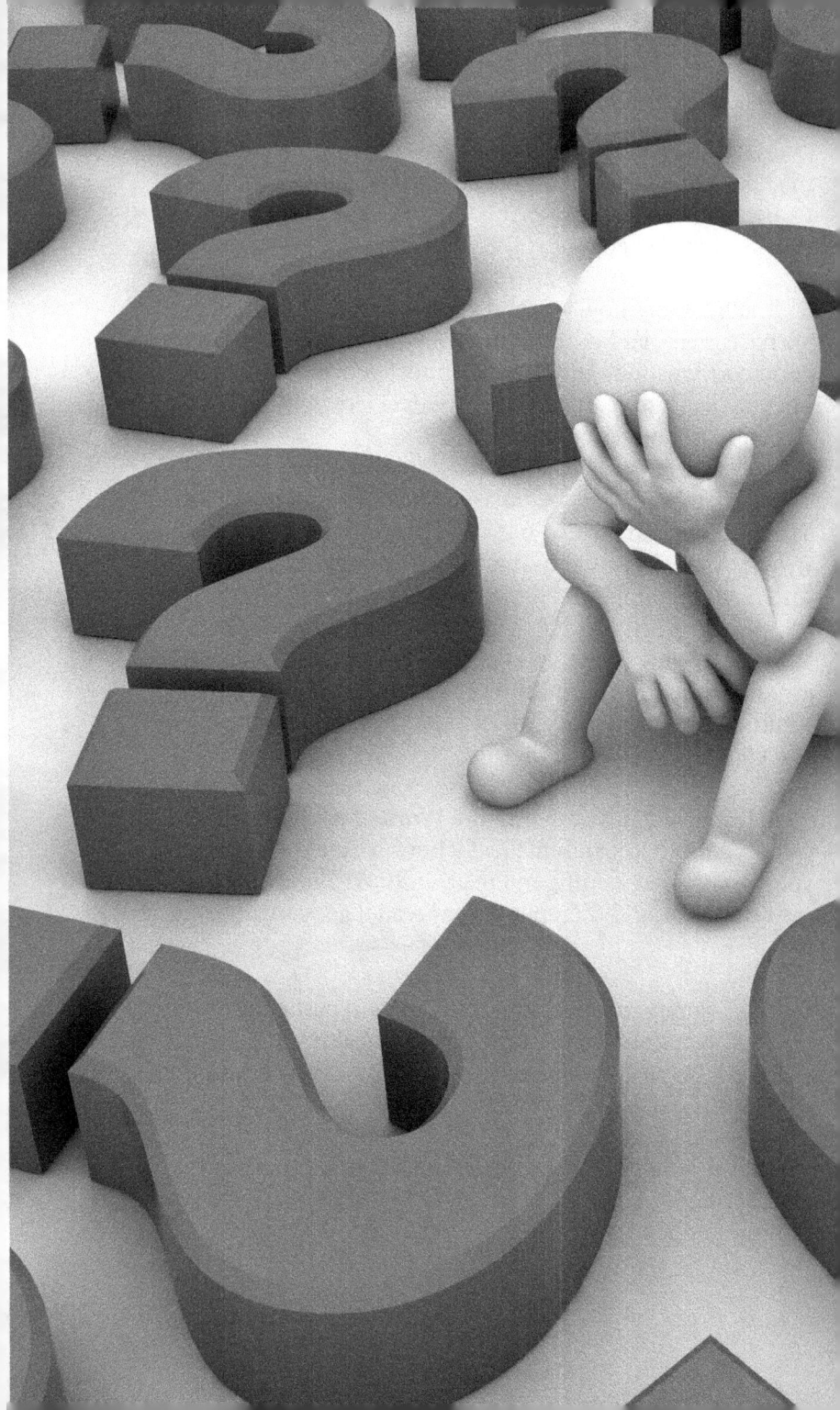

CONCLUSION:
ASK FOR HELP

There are a lot of things that I haven't been very good at for most of my life.

One of the first things that comes to mind, though, is that I've never been very good at asking for help. I've always thought that if I asked for help, then I would be imposing on people, and I never wanted to do that.

It's taken me most of my life to realize that not only do I need help, but that by not asking for or accepting help, I was pushing people away. Since I've learned to ask for help, I've received more than I could ever repay, and yet everyone has given me help without any desire for repayment.

It's that same view that you need to take with your family. It doesn't matter if it's your husband, wife, partner, son, daughter, or anybody else. You need their help, and if you ask in the right way, they will jump at the chance to help you.

It's hard enough to make big changes to your diet and lifestyle, and it's even harder to stick to them. If you refuse the help of your family and friends just because you "believe" that they're not going to be willing to help you, then you've made your own journey so much harder. And you've essentially cut off the possibility that you'll be able one day to help them also change their own health when they might need it.

I truly hope that this book can help you on your journey toward greater health and happiness. And just like your family, I'm also willing to help. It's what makes my job and my life meaningful and better. If you have questions or just want to say hello, please email me at jeremy@jeremyhendon.com. I may not always reply the same day (I get behind on emails just like everybody else), but I promise that I'll reply as soon as possible.

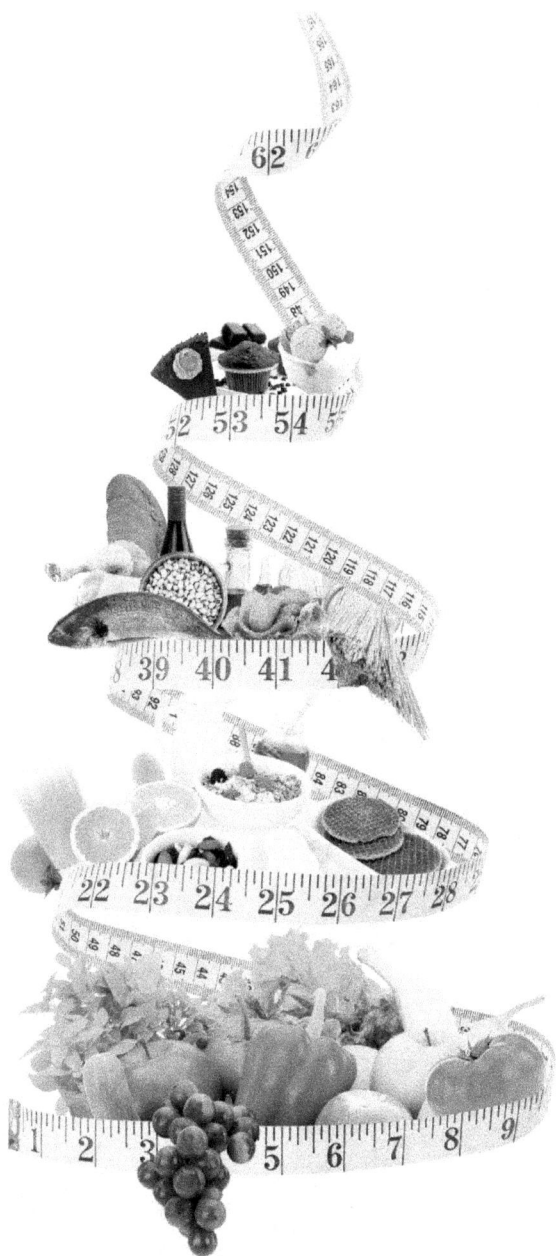

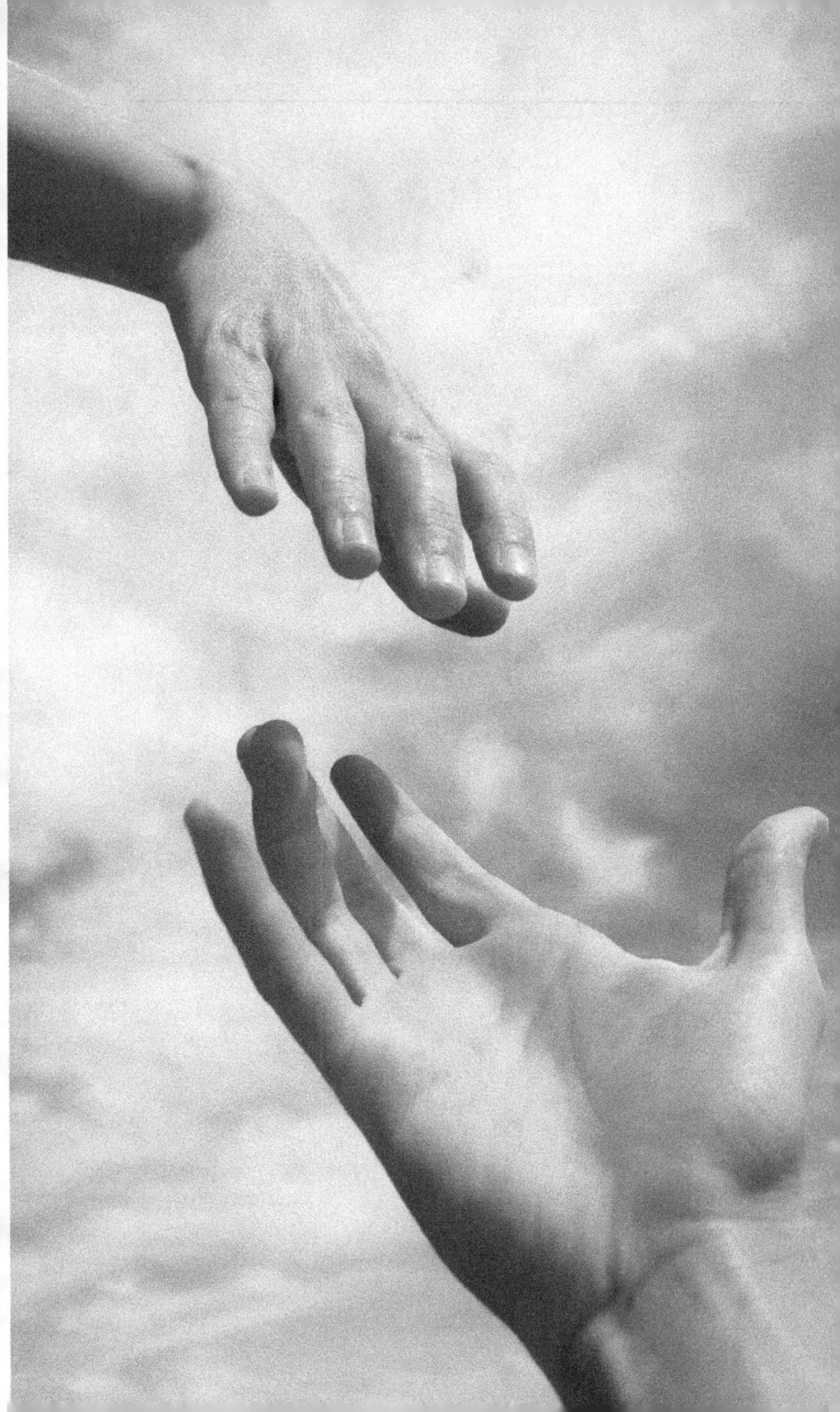

CHEAT SHEET— GETTING THE SUPPORT OF YOUR FAMILY AND FRIENDS

This is a quick and easy tool to use any time you need to figure out how to best gain the support, encouragement, and involvement of a family member or friend.

Use a separate cheat sheet for each person (you can print copies of the cheat sheet online by going to: http://jeremyhendon.com/cheat-sheet).

STEP #1: BELIEVE IN YOUR GOLDEN OPPORTUNITY.

Action Step: A 10 minute exercise - Write down as many reasons as possible that changing your diet and getting healthier will *benefit* both you AND your family.

_____

_____

_____

_____

_____

_____

_____

_____

_____

_____

_____

_____

_____

_____

_____

STEP #2: HOW CAN YOUR FAMILY HELP YOU?

Action Step: Another 10-minute exercise - Write down as many ways as possible that your family could potentially **help** you stick to your diet and get healthier.

_____

_____

_____

_____

_____

_____

_____

_____

_____

_____

_____

_____

_____

_____

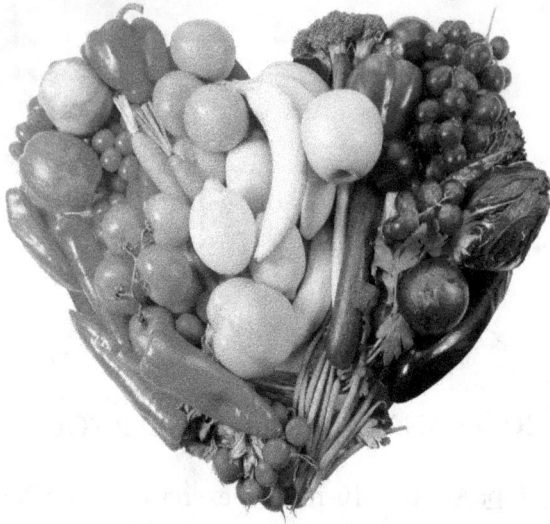

STEP #3: TALK TO YOUR FAMILY.

Action Step: Have a "Can You Help Me Win?" Conversation. Use the scripts below for guidance.

1. Start the conversation with a question, and actually wait for a reply.
    a. "Do you have time to talk?"
    b. "Do you have a minute?"
    c. "Can I ask you about something?"

2. Tell them your goal, why it's important, and that you want their help.
    a. "I would like to lose 20 lbs in the next 3 months so that I can start feeling better every day, and I'd love your help."
    b. "I want to stick a Paleo diet for the next month. It's really important to me because I've been feeling really tired and sick. I think you could really help me with this."

3. Tell them why they'd be great at helping you.
 a. "You've always been so good at sticking to anything you start. I feel like you could help me learn how to do that better."
 b. "Sometimes I don't have the best attitude toward things like this, but you're always so positive and encouraging that I think you could really help me succeed."

4. Ask if they're willing to help and if they have any thoughts.
 a. "What do you think?"
 b. "How does that plan sound to you?"

5. Ask for specific ideas they have to help you reach your goals.
 a. "What do you think might be the best way to help me stick to this diet?
 b. "Do you have any thoughts or suggestions for how you could help me?"

6. Adapt the ways they can help you. There are no scripts for this. At this point in the conversation, you need to listen to their suggestions and actually work with them to come up with ways that they can help, even if those ways are small at first. Just getting them involved is a step in the right direction.

7. Set an expectation for future conversations and for check-ins.
 a. "I'd love to have you ask me at the end of every day how I've done, so that I can be more accountable."
 b. "This has been so helpful, and I'm really excited. Do you think we could chat about it again in a week to see how I'm doing and if you have any other thoughts or suggestions?"

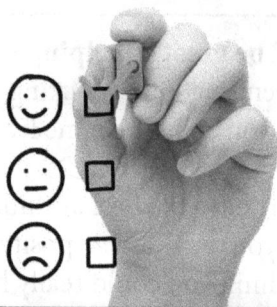

SPECIAL REQUEST

Please Review This Book on Amazon!

Amazon.com and word of mouth are how most people hear about books today.

If you liked this book, then please help me reach more people by either telling a friend about my book or leaving me a review on Amazon.

Just visit Amazon.com and search for the title of this book.

Image Attributions

www.ingramcontent.com/pod-product-compliance
Lightning Source LLC
Chambersburg PA
CBHW070850280326
41934CB00008B/1386